SAFETY EDUCATION

man, his machines,
and his environment

SAFETY EDUCATION
man, his machines, and his environment

W. WAYNE WORICK

*Professor and Coordinator
of Health and Safety Education,
Chicago State University*

PRENTICE-HALL, INC., Englewood Cliffs, New Jersey

Library of Congress Cataloging in Publication Data

WORICK, W   WAYNE, DATE
   Safety education.

   Includes bibliographies.
   1. Safety education.   2. Accidents, Prevention.
3. Safety education, Industrial. I. Title.
HV675.W63   613.8'07   74-20663
ISBN 0-13-785683-0

Printed in the United States of America

10 9 8 7 6 5 4 3 2 1

PRENTICE-HALL INTERNATIONAL, INC., *London*
PRENTICE-HALL OF AUSTRALIA, PTY. LTD., *Sydney*
PRENTICE-HALL OF CANADA, LTD., *Toronto*
PRENTICE-HALL OF INDIA PRIVATE LIMITED, *New Delhi*
PRENTICE-HALL OF JAPAN, INC., *Tokyo*

to Marion Taylor,
who made it happen

contents

foreword

As long as accidents continue to be the leading cause of death among children and youth there will be a continuing need for improved and expanded safety education in our schools and colleges.

Unfortunately there is no Salk vaccine for accidents. Nor is there a ground swell of demand from an outraged public, as there would be if an epidemic swept the land. Yet accidents *are* an epidemic, taking an ever growing toll of our human, physical, and financial resources.

No, there is no panacea; no magic amulet to ward off the accident demon.

But there is a cure, and the schools can—indeed, must—play a major role in that cure, by teaching their students from kindergarten through college, that accidents *can* be prevented, that the consequences of accidents can be lessened.

Dr. Worick's book provides a significant aid in the cure, by providing teacher training institutions with another tool for the safety education of the embryonic teacher and safety professional. School and college teachers and administrators will also find it helpful in expanding their own background in safety.

The author is to be commended for his contribution to the safety movement.

Vincent L. Tofany
President
National Safety Council

preface

Safety Education: Man, His Machines and His Environment is designed primarily for use in safety and safety education courses at the college level. However, industrial supervisors, fleet supervisors, school administrators, high school and higher education safety teachers will also find the book a useful addition to their libraries. The book discusses many causes of accidents and covers the major areas of safety such as traffic, fire, school, industry, farming, recreation, and the home. Suggested countermeasures against accidents are included in each section. The book is based on the premise that accidents are the result of either unsafe acts, unsafe conditions, or both, and that to prevent them man must interact safely with his machines and his environment.

This book recognizes that the universe is a system composed of many subsystems. When something goes wrong in one of the systems, the stage is set for a possible accident. We must consider the whole system in which the accident occurred, not just the accident itself, if we are to reduce accidents to a minimum. Sample task analyses can be found in several different parts of the text.

The central theme is that accidents can be prevented and that needless deaths through accidents are a betrayal to our society. The book recognizes accidents as a major health problem, having a pervasive negative impact upon our society by prematurely terminating the lives of so many people, especially the young.

Any errors found in the book are mine and not those of the reviewers. Your comments will be welcome and all suggestions will be given serious consideration in future revisions.

All textbooks require contributions from many sources and this one is no exception. A special thanks to all of the following people and organizations who made such valuable contributions to this book: Mr. Vincent Tofany, President of the National Safety Council, for writing the stimulating foreword; Dr. Forrest Hazard, Attorney at Law and English Professor at Chicago State University, for reviewing the entire book and for his many helpful suggestions in preparing the chapter on legal responsibility in school safety; Wm. Fletcher and Wm. Hanford, Agricultural Engineers, National Safety Council, for reviewing the chapter on farm safety and for preparing the "Task Analysis of the Combine Operation"; Ken Licht, Manager, School and College Department, Jack Green, Sr., Assistant Manager, School and College Department, and Barbara Rowder, Staff Representative, Driver Education, of the National Safety Council for their many suggestions and editorial comments; Dr. Gerald Driessen, Senior Research Scientist, National Safety Council, for reviewing Chapter 2; Dr. George Oberle, Chairman, Department of Health, Physical Education, Recreation and Athletics, Chicago State University, for his guidance and patience; Dr. David Rogers, Hockey Coach, Chicago State University, for his many editorial comments on sports safety; Marion Taylor, Library Science Department, Chicago State University, for her review of many chapters and editorial comments; Robert Borkenstein, eminent authority on alcohol and driving, Indiana University, for his help with the section on alcohol and driving; Jeanne Vitale, a student of mine, for her many editorial comments and for designing Figure 3–1; Edward Johnson, Director, Safety Education, Illinois State Supt. of Instruction, for reviewing Chapters 9 and 10 on school safety and safety education; Dr. W. Laurance Quane, Illinois State University, for reviewing Chapter 1 and designing Figure 1–1; Ruth Hammersmith, Librarian, National Safety Council, who made this book possible by making the facilities of the National Safety Council Library available to me and locating many valuable references; and last but not least Mary Swanson, Chicago State University, for her excellent job of typing the manuscript.

W. WAYNE WORICK

SAFETY EDUCATION
man, his machines,
and his environment

1

a philosophy of safety and safety education

Through philosophy man searches for truth, for the reasons for things. He uses philosophy to develop his goals, his objectives, and the underlying principles that guide his life. His philosophy of life cannot be separated from his philosophy of safety, since both have to do with his values. Man must understand and believe that he has a responsibility to himself and to others to preserve human life and resources. It is simply the right thing to do.

Safety touches many areas of man's life. There are ethical, moral, religious, aesthetic, legal, and many other considerations that involve safety.

To function at full capacity man must preserve his health. From an ethical standpoint man owes it to himself and those who depend upon him to preserve his health in order to function at his best, and he owes it to all persons to be considerate of their lives, limbs, and possessions.[1]

Man's moral and spiritual beliefs contribute to his sense of values and thus help safeguard his behavior.[2] Since in our society man has the fundamental right to be free from the wrongful acts of others, there are legal implications to unsafe behavior.

A positive relationship exists among all the values that a person

[1] H. H. Horne, Reprint of "A Philosophy of Safety and Safety Education," *Safety Education Digest* (New York: Center for Safety Education, New York University), June 1940, p. 1.
[2] Horne, "Philosophy of Safety," p. 2.

1

holds; his personal values of safety consciousness are related to the values he shows in social responsibility, citizenship, and morality. We must therefore build proper safety values into everyone's philosophy of life.[3]

Man's progress depends to a large extent on his safety. At the same time, that progress is admittedly dependent upon taking risks. Therefore, it is not the function of safety and safety education to stop man from taking risks for either progress or enjoyment. Rather, the risks must be minimized to attain maximum progress. Our space program is a good example of how man takes risks to advance technology and create a better life. At the same time, every precaution possible is taken to ensure that the space pioneers return safely.

Herbert J. Stack and J. Duke Elkow expressed this philosophy well when they said:

> Civilized man constantly strives to improve his condition to enjoy a more plentiful life, and he can accomplish this only through persistent untiring efforts. The philosophy of safety humanizes science as it contributes to the life and welfare of mankind.[4]

SAFETY AND SAFETY EDUCATION DEFINED

Workers in the field of accident prevention have struggled for years to find a definition of "safety" that would be widely accepted. Some of the definitions that have been offered are very narrow and some very broad. One element, however, is common to them all: safety does involve the conservation of human resources and materials. In addition, some people would include the word "security" in a definition of safety, reflecting the legitimate concern of being safe from robbers, vandals, and other wrongdoers. Others would include "health" as a major factor and therefore would include health education as a part of safety education, or vice versa. We would not argue with either of these views, but since our primary concern is for the prevention of accidents, we have chosen the following definition: **"Safety is the minimization of injury and loss resulting from nondeliberate acts such as accidents and natural calamities."** [5] This definition is compatible with our definition of an accident as that occurrence in a sequence of events that usually produces unintended injury, death, or property damage (see Chapter 2). Furthermore, this definition of safety helps to define our goal: to prevent those events

---

[3] Marland K. Strasser, J. E. Aaron, R. C. Bohn, and J. R. Eales, *Fundamentals of Safety Education*, 2nd ed. (New York: The Macmillan Company, 1973), p. 69.

[4] Herbert J. Stack and J. Duke Elkow, *Education for Safe Living*, 4th ed. (Englewood Cliffs, N. J.: Prentice-Hall, Inc., © 1966), p. 14.

[5] National Safety Council, "Safety, What Is It?" *School Safety World Newsletter*, Summer 1973.

unplanned or unpremeditated that result in injury, loss of life, or destruction of property.

Safety education is a means by which we reach our goal. It is the way to establish safe behavior. Just as for the word "safety," there are many definitions of "safety education," depending upon one's goals and purposes. We have chosen the following: **Safety education is the sum of experiences that favorably affects the development of habits, skills, attitudes, and knowledges conducive to safe behavior.**

A breakdown of our definition may help to clarify it. The "sum of experiences" suggests that safety education must come from many sources and that it begins at birth and continues throughout life. Figure 1-1 illustrates the great variety of safety education sources that a person is exposed to before, during, and after his educational years.

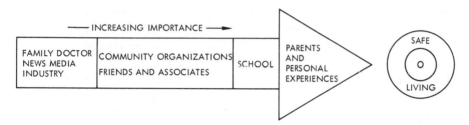

Figure 1-1. *Sources of safety education. Diagram design courtesy of W. Laurance Quane.*

The second part of our definition concerns the development of habits, skills, attitudes, and knowledges conducive to safe behavior. If an experience does not have a favorable effect on these factors, it is not safety education, but rather a deterrent to it. Through various media and our associations with people, we are constantly exposed to much information concerning health and safety' that is not based on scientific evidence. Yet it is of primary importance to be able to distinguish the safe from the unsafe. Many children, for instance, because of exposure to improper safety techniques and attitudes by the media, parents, and others, are slow in developing safe behavior.

SHARED RESPONSIBILITY FOR SAFETY EDUCATION

A person's total safety education, as we know, originates from several sources. But how viable are these sources in contributing to satisfactory safety education?

Obviously a child's safety education must begin in the home, since it is there that he is first exposed to safety hazards. Parents shoulder the main responsibility for the safety and safety education of the child in his early years.

Many children do receive fine safety training in the home, but home safety programs generally tend to be weak, as evidenced by the number of home accidents. Bad safety practices run rampant in many homes simply because people are not properly trained in safe living practices and do not hold attitudes conducive to safety. Frequently it is only after an accident occurs that one becomes aware of an unsafe act or condition. To make matters worse, children tend to model their behavior after their parents and other members of the family. As a result, much of a child's early safety education can be decompensating.

To a large extent, early safety education involves "avoidance conditioning," resulting, for example, from pain after touching a hot, cold, or sharp object. Although the influence of the home in safety education will diminish somewhat after the child starts school, much of his education, nevertheless, will continue to be rooted in the home environment for years to come. This fact alone makes it important to improve our home, as well as our school, safety programs.

Another source of safety education may be counselling by the family doctor, who is probably well grounded in fundamentals of safety. But since a doctor's time is very limited, obviously we cannot rely on the medical profession through counselling to be a major source of safety education for our youth.

There are many community organizations, such as the YMCA or YWCA, Girl Scouts, Boy Scouts, Red Cross, and others, that have some personnel on their staffs capable of giving safety instruction, most of which will relate directly to recreation. Such programs are limited, however, because these organizations have neither the facilities nor the staffs to accommodate hundreds of individuals in a comprehensive program such as safety education.

Safety has been discussed through the news media, and the immediate effects have often been good. However, the effects are not long lasting, and the number of persons reached is limited. Perhaps the most advanced and continuous safety education efforts have come from industry. Companies make valuable contributions to safety education among their workers, as well as in programs through the schools. However, industry cannot assume the responsibility for safety education for the entire community.

Churches represent a source of safety education. Through their spiritual and moral teachings, they contribute heavily to safety values, and the aims and objectives of safety education are most compatible with the teachings of religion. But the churches lack the staffs necessary for such a task, and church attendance is not sufficient to reach the millions of children who need this education.

Considering all the possible sources of safety education in a community, the schools represent the only place with the potential for adequate personnel and facilities, plus access to millions of young children in a semi-captive audience. Therefore, the schools must bear a major share of responsibility for the safety education of our children. This educational process should be well planned, well organized, and properly budgeted. Safety education must start on the day the child enters school and must continue throughout his school career, for school safety education lays the foundation for the continuing safety education that takes place throughout life. Teacher education institutions need to step up their efforts to provide teachers at all levels equipped to handle safety education in the schools.

The responsibility for safety education then is shared, with the major portion taking place in the home and in the schools. Ideally the efforts of all community agencies should be coordinated with those of the school and the home.

Through experience we know that most accidents are caused by human error or unsafe acts. We must find out why these acts take place and correct the situation through education and technology. The development of proper safety habits, attitudes, knowledges, and skills represents the best opportunity for making significant inroads into the accident problem. Technology will help, but in the end the individual must react correctly to hazardous situations. He must be educated to recognize hazards, evaluate them, remove them, or compensate for them.

H. H. Horne succinctly described the function of safety and safety education when he said:

> Safety education aims to make the physical survival of a person possible. As such it is a means to all the good ends of life. Its great contribution is in delivering the person whole so that the other agencies of the good life may make the personality wholesome. Safety education is not an end in itself; it is a means to all good ends. It takes you where you are going so that you arrive; it protects you while you are there; and then it brings you back so you may go again. We believe in safety because we believe in life.[6]

SOCIAL IMPLICATIONS OF ACCIDENTS

Accidents are one of the critical social and public health issues of our time. They are the leading cause of death in the age group 1–38.[7] Any problem or phenomenon that strikes in such a devastating manner at

---

[6] Horne, "Philosophy of Safety," p. 2.
[7] National Safety Council, *Accident Facts 1973 Edition* (Chicago, 1973), p. 9.

people in so young an age group must be considered one of our major, if not our foremost, public health problems. Special interest groups comment on ecology, the drug issue, the effects of disease, the welfare problem—admittedly all great concerns—but these same groups rarely mention accidents in their discussions and prognostications.

A college dean turns down a federally supported driver education program with the comment, "So what if we are killing 56,000 people a year in automobile accidents?" A school board refuses to support driver education. This lack of concern about a very real and pressing public health problem is a sad commentary upon our society.

The actual social implications of accidents are so immense that they defy accurate description. A young doctor, scientist, teacher, lawyer, or engineer has his or her life snuffed out in a matter of seconds in a flaming automobile crash or some other accident. Could one of these have been another Einstein or Curie in the offing? Could one of these individuals have discovered some form of hydrogen or thermal energy to benefit mankind? And even if the victim was merely competent at his or her job, the loss is tragic.

Normally secure family members can have their hopes, desires, and security, as well as their whole lives, rearranged because of an accident. They may in turn become a financial burden upon society, to say nothing of the pain, anguish, and suffering they endure, and the valuable services lost to the community.

We are killing an average of 13 people per hour in the United States, and injuring 1,310 during the same period.[8] The average hourly cost of these deaths is an estimated $4,500,000—more than $70,000 per minute. How long will society continue to tolerate this waste? Ironically, most of these accidents could have been prevented.

In 1972 we had approximately 117,000 accidental deaths and an estimated 11,500,000 disabling injuries in the United States.[9] These accidents and disabling injuries occur as isolated events in every part of the nation. Yet, they fail to arouse public concern.

Total death figures present only part of the picture. To understand the pervasive negative impact of accidental deaths upon society, consider deaths versus age. For example, leading disease killers such as cancer and heart disease tend to strike more people in their later years. Accidents tend to involve more of the younger population. Therefore, a sudden cure for the accident problem would have a much more dramatic effect on the total life span than would a sudden cure for cancer or heart disease. But people rarely consider accidents in this light. Accidents continue year after year with the same end results, while a disease striking with equal

[8] National Safety Council, *Accident Facts 1973*, p. 11.
[9] National Safety Council, *Accident Facts 1973*, p. 3.

devastation would undoubtedly trigger a massive research program. It is not that it is somehow more acceptable to have people die of cancer or heart disease, but simply that so many accidents need not happen at all.

Table 1-1 shows how accidents rank as a cause of death among persons of all ages (based on official figures for 1969). Table 1-2 shows the principal classes of accidental deaths from 1903 to 1972. Table 1-3 illustrates the economic implications of accidents. These tables have been grouped at the end of the chapter for convenience; they evidence the serious nature of the accident problem.

SUMMARY

Humanitarian as well as economic considerations dictate that our society become aroused and demand immediate action to minimize the accident problem. Man will continue to take risks in the interest of progress. That progress will bring new hazards with which he must cope. But he must evaluate his risks, eliminate those he can, and compensate for or control those he cannot eliminate. Failure to do so will allow accidents to continue to plague our society.

Our goal in safety and safety education is to reduce accidents to an irreducible minimum. Although some accidents do occur by chance alone, the overwhelming majority of accidents can be and should be prevented.

Through safety and safety education we can create both a public consciousness and a better public philosophy of safety. As Horne said, "We believe in safety because we believe in life." Needless deaths through accidents are a betrayal of our society.

Table 1-1. Accidents versus other causes of death.

Cause	Number of Deaths			Death Rates*		
	Total	Male	Female	Total	Male	Female
All Causes....................	1,921,990	1,080,926	841,064	954	1,103	814
Heart disease......................	739,265	421,845	317,420	367	430	307
Cancer............................	323,092	176,142	146,950	160	180	142
Stroke (cerebrovascular disease)......	207,179	94,227	112,952	103	96	109
Accidents........................	**116,385**	**80,706**	**35,679**	**58**	**82**	**35**
Motor-vehicle....	55,791	40,213	15,578	28	41	15
Pneumonia.........................	62,394	34,852	27,542	31	36	27
Diabetes mellitus...................	38,541	15,689	22,852	19	16	22
Arteriosclerosis....................	33,063	14,346	18,717	16	15	18

*Deaths per 100,000 population.

Reproduced from Accident Facts 1973 Edition, *p. 9, courtesy of the National Safety Council.*

Table 1-2. Principal classes of accidental deaths, 1903 to 1972.

Year	TOTAL§ Deaths	Rate†	Motor-Vehicle Deaths	Rate†	Work Deaths	Rate†	Home Deaths	Rate†	Public Non-Motor-Vehicle Deaths	Rate†
1903-1907 ave......	72,400	88.9	400	0.5	**		**		**	
1908-1912 ave......	74,900	83.1	1,900	2.1	**		**		**	
1913..............	82,500	85.5	4,200	4.4	**		**		**	
1914..............	77,000	78.6	4,700	4.8	**		**		**	
1915..............	76,200	76.7	6,600	6.6	**		**		**	
1916..............	84,800	84.1	8,200	8.1	**		**		**	
1917..............	90,100	88.2	10,200	10.0	**		**		**	
1918..............	85,100	82.1	10,700	10.3	**		**		**	
1919..............	75,500	71.9	11,200	10.7	**		**		**	
1920..............	75,900	71.2	12,500	11.7	**		**		**	
1921..............	74,000	68.4	13,900	12.9	**		**		**	
1922..............	76,300	69.4	15,300	13.9	**		**		**	
1923..............	84,400	75.7	18,400	16.5	**		**		**	
1924..............	85,600	75.6	19,400	17.1	**		**		**	
1925..............	90,000	78.4	21,900	19.1	**		**		**	
1926..............	91,700	78.7	23,400	20.1	**		**		**	
1927..............	92,700	78.4	25,800	21.8	**		**		**	
1928..............	95,000	79.3	28,000	23.4	19,000	15.8	30,000	24.9	21,000	17.4
1929..............	98,200	80.8	31,200	25.7	20,000	16.4	30,000	24.6	20,000	16.4
1930..............	99,100	80.5	32,900	26.7	19,000	15.4	30,000	24.4	20,000	16.3
1931..............	97,300	78.5	33,700	27.2	17,500	14.1	29,000	23.4	20,000	16.1
1932..............	89,000	71.3	29,500	23.6	15,000	12.0	29,000	23.2	18,000	14.4
1933..............	90,932	72.4	31,363	25.0	14,500	11.6	29,500	23.5	18,500	14.7
1934..............	100,977	79.9	36,101	28.6	16,000	12.7	34,000	26.9	18,000	14.2
1935..............	99,773	78.4	36,369	28.6	16,500	13.0	32,000	25.2	18,000	14.2
1936..............	110,052	85.9	38,089	29.7	18,500	14.5	37,000	28.9	19,500	15.2
1937..............	105,205	81.7	39,643	30.8	19,000	14.8	32,000	24.8	18,000	14.0
1938..............	93,805	72.3	32,582	25.1	16,000	12.3	31,000	23.9	17,000	13.1
1939..............	92,623	70.8	32,386	24.7	15,500	11.8	31,000	23.7	16,000	12.2
1940..............	96,885	73.4	34,501	26.1	17,000	12.9	31,500	23.9	16,500	12.5
1941..............	101,513	76.3	39,969	30.0	18,000	13.5	30,000	22.5	16,500	12.4
1942..............	95,889	71.6	28,309	21.1	18,500	13.8	30,500	22.8	16,000	12.0
1943..............	99,038	73.8	23,823	17.8	17,500	13.0	33,500	25.0	17,000	12.7
1944..............	95,237	71.7	24,282	18.3	16,000	12.0	32,500	24.5	16,000	12.0
1945..............	95,918	72.4	28,076	21.2	16,500	12.5	33,500	25.3	16,000	12.1
1946..............	98,033	70.0	33,411	23.9	16,500	11.8	33,000	23.6	17,500	12.5
1947..............	99,579	69.4	32,697	22.8	17,000	11.9	34,500	24.1	18,000	12.6
1948 (5th Revn.)††..	98,001	67.1	32,259	22.1	16,000	11.0	35,000	24.0	17,000	11.6
1948 (6th Revn.)††..	93,000	63.7	32,259	22.1	16,000	11.0	31,000	21.2	16,000	11.0
1949..............	90,106	60.6	31,701	21.3	15,000	10.1	31,000	20.9	15,000	10.1
1950..............	91,249	60.3	34,763	23.0	15,500	10.2	29,000	19.2	15,000	9.9
1951..............	95,871	62.5	36,996	24.1	16,000	10.4	30,000	19.6	16,000	10.4
1952..............	96,172	61.8	37,794	24.3	15,000	9.6	30,500	19.6	16,000	10.3
1953..............	95,032	60.1	37,955	24.0	15,000	9.5	29,000	18.3	16,500	10.4
1954..............	90,032	55.9	35,586	22.1	14,000	8.7	28,000	17.4	15,500	9.6
1955..............	93,443	56.9	38,426	23.4	14,200	8.6	28,500	17.3	15,500	9.4
1956..............	94,780	56.6	39,628	23.7	14,300	8.5	28,000	16.7	16,000	9.6
1957..............	95,307	55.9	38,702	22.7	14,200	8.3	28,000	16.4	17,500	10.3
1958..............	90,604	52.3	36,981	21.3	13,300	7.7	26,500	15.3	16,500	9.5
1959..............	92,080	52.2	37,910	21.5	13,800	7.8	27,000	15.3	16,500	9.3
1960..............	93,806	52.1	38,137	21.2	13,800	7.7	28,000	15.6	17,000	9.4
1961..............	92,249	50.4	38,091	20.8	13,500	7.4	27,000	14.8	16,500	9.0
1962..............	97,139	52.3	40,804	22.0	13,700	7.4	28,500	15.3	17,000	9.2
1963..............	100,669	53.4	43,564	23.1	14,200	7.5	28,500	15.1	17,500	9.3
1964..............	105,000	54.9	47,700	25.0	14,200	7.4	28,000	14.6	18,500	9.7
1965..............	108,004	55.8	49,163	25.4	14,100	7.3	28,500	14.7	19,500	10.1
1966..............	113,563	58.1	53,041	27.1	14,500	7.4	29,500	15.1	20,000	10.2
1967..............	113,169	57.3	52,924	26.8	14,200	7.2	29,000	14.7	20,500	10.4
1968..............	114,864	57.6	54,862	27.5	14,300	7.2	28,000	14.0	21,500	10.8
1969..............	116,385	57.8	55,791	27.7	14,300	7.1	27,500	13.7	22,500	11.2
1970..............	115,000	56.4	54,800	26.9	14,300	7.0	27,000	13.2	22,500	11.0
1971..............	115,000	55.8	54,700	26.5	14,200	6.9	27,500	13.3	22,500	10.9
1972..............	117,000	56.2	56,600	27.2	14,100	6.8	27,000	13.0	23,500	11.3
Changes										
1962 to 1972........	+20%	+7%	+39%	+24%	+3%	−8%	−5%	−15%	+38%	+23%
1971 to 1972........	+ 2%	+1%	+ 3%	+ 3%	−1%	−1%	−2%	− 2%	+ 4%	+ 4%

Source: Total deaths and motor-vehicle deaths from 1903 to 1932 calculated from National Center for Health Statistics data for death registration states; from 1933 to 1948 (5th Revn.), 1949 to 1963, 1965 to 1969 they are NCHS totals for the United States. All other figures are National Safety Council estimates based on data from NCHS, state and city vital statistics departments and other sources.

§Duplications between Motor-Vehicle, Work and Home are eliminated in the TOTAL column.

†Rates are deaths per 100,000 population.   **Data insufficient to estimate yearly totals.

††In 1948, a revision was made in the official method of classification, the International List of Causes of Death. In the table, the first figures for 1948 are comparable with those for earlier years; the second figures are comparable with those for later years.

Reproduced from Accident Facts 1973 Edition, *p. 13, courtesy of the National Safety Council.*

Table 1-3. Costs of accidents in 1972 *—$37.0 billion.

These costs include: (billion)

Wage losses due to temporary inability to work, lower wages after returning to work due to permanent impairment, present value of future earnings lost by those totally incapacitated or killed $12.0

Medical fees, hospital expenses .... $ 3.9

Insurance administrative and claim settlement costs (claims are not identified separately but losses for which claim payments are made are included in other items in this table—see note below) .... $ 7.6

Property damage in motor-vehicle accidents .... $ 6.0

Property destroyed by fire .... $ 2.3

Money value of time lost by workers other than those with disabling injuries, who are directly or indirectly involved in accidents .... $ 5.2

Notes on certain accident costs

There are alternative ways of identifying certain costs of accidents. The items in the table above represent one of the ways. All measurable costs have been included, and none have been included twice. See comments below under insurance costs.

Wage losses. Loss of productivity by injured or killed workers is a loss to the nation. Since, theoretically, a worker's contribution to the wealth of the nation is measured in terms of wages, then the sum total of wages lost due to accidents provides a measure of this lost productivity. For nonfatal injuries, actual wage losses are used; for fatalities and permanently disabling injuries, the figure used is the present value of all future earnings lost.

Insurance administrative and claim settlement costs. This is the difference between premiums paid *to* insurance companies and claims paid *by* them; it is their cost of doing business and is a part of the accident cost total. *Claims* paid by insurance companies are not identified separately in the total. Since every claim is paid to a claimant for such losses as wages, medical and hospital expense, etc., losses for which claims are paid are already included in various items in the table.

*Costs are not comparable with previous years. As additional or more precise data become available they are used from that year forward, but previously estimated figures are not revised.

Reproduced from Accident Facts 1973 Edition, *p. 4, courtesy of the National Safety Council.*

SUGGESTED STUDENT ACTIVITIES

1. Devise a definition of safety and safety education.
2. Compare the economic costs of accidents with those of education, medical care, and others.
3. Survey your community to determine what agencies are making safety and safety education efforts.
4. Compare graphically accidents and diseases for three different age groups.
5. Write a paper on your philosophy of safety and safety education.

BIBLIOGRAPHY

HORNE, H. H. Reprint of "A Philosophy of Safety and Safety Education." *Safety Education Digest* (New York: Center for Safety Education, New York University), June 1940, pp. 1–2.

NATIONAL SAFETY COUNCIL. *Accident Facts 1973 Edition.* Chicago, 1973.

NATIONAL SAFETY COUNCIL. "Safety, What Is It?" *School Safety World Newsletter,* Summer 1973.

STACK, HERBERT J., and ELKOW, J. DUKE. *Education for Safe Living.* 4th ed. Englewood Cliffs, N. J.: Prentice-Hall, Inc., 1966.

STRASSER, MARLAND K.; AARON, J. E.; BOHN, R. C.; and EALES, J. R. *Fundamentals of Safety Education.* 2nd ed. New York: The Macmillan Company, 1973.

2

using accident data

The use of accident data and statistics can be considered a science in itself. Therefore, a specialist working in the field of accident prevention needs a basic foundation in their proper use. He should research the subject thoroughly and expose himself to both basic and advanced courses in the use of statistics.

Accident statistics have a complexity and massiveness that are at times overwhelming, even to the highly experienced investigator. All too often he misinterprets these statistics because he does not understand their meaning, or because he bases his conclusions on insufficient data. Another common pitfall is the attempt to apply abstract psychological theories to accident data. (See Chapter 3 on Accident Proneness.) Accident data can be utilized in many different ways, and can be very effective if properly applied within the context of their limitations. However, such statistics should always be used with caution, and the limitations of any conclusions drawn from specific data should be carefully explained.

Lack of valid accident data is a major stumbling block in all phases of accident prevention. It retards both the development of more sophisticated machinery and improvement in the safety of human behavior. The importance of this data cannot be overemphasized.

Accident data must be collected on a very thorough and systematic basis, completely analyzed, revalidated, applied in accident prevention programs, reevaluated, and then reapplied. The history of industrial safety programs indicates that once this process is accomplished in all areas, there will be more hope for a significant reduction in all accidental deaths, injuries, and property damage losses.

Adequate accident data, if properly utilized, should provide more definitive answers regarding the causes of accidents and their interrelationships. This would allow us to make maximum use of the latest "systems" engineering techniques to produce machinery and equipment that could be operated with maximum safety and efficiency. It would also enable us to develop educational techniques and programs to teach people how to interact safely with machinery and the rest of their environment.

DEFINITION OF AN ACCIDENT

In the United States the most widely accepted definition of an accident is the one used by the National Safety Council: **"that occurrence in a sequence of events which usually produces unintended injury, death or property damage."** [1]

The first part of the definition—that an accident is "that occurrence in a sequence of events"—recognizes that there are several different events occurring that lead up to the "occurrence," or accident, which produces injury, death, or property damage. This suggests, and we agree, that there are multiple causes or variables with all accidents.

The phrase "which usually produces unintended injury, death, or property damage" implies that if the sequence of events leading to the injury, death, or property damage is purposely planned or promoted, then the result is not an accident. For example, an injury received by the victim of a robbery would not be considered an accident since the robbery was premeditated.

This definition of an accident recognizes that death, injury, or property damage is the terminal event in the entire sequence. It also implies that an interruption in the sequence of events could prevent the accident.

DEATH AND INJURY RATES

There are many problems in determining death and injury rates. For example, in order to be classified as death from an accident, the death must occur within one year from the date of the accident and must be the result of accident-related causes. One can readily see that even death

---

[1] National Safety Council, *Accident Facts 1973 Edition* (Chicago, 1973), p. 97.

statistics can never be absolutely accurate, but modern diagnostic techniques do provide a reasonable degree of accuracy.

Injury statistics tend to be even more nebulous than death statistics, for two reasons. First, minor injuries tend not to be reported; thus many never show up in statistics. However, they are often estimated, hopefully with some accuracy. Second, the definition of an injury varies from person to person and from organization to organization. For example, the National Safety Council uses the term "disabling injury" in its reporting. It defines a disabling injury as one that prevents a person from performing any of his or her usual activities for a full day beyond the day of the accident. The Council has adopted this definition for injuries in all categories.

In contrast, the National Health Survey breaks its definition of injury into two categories—bed disabling injuries and restricted activity injuries. It defines a bed disabling injury as one that confines a person to bed for more than half of the daylight hours (on the day of the accident or some of the following day). A restricted activity injury is defined as one that causes a person to cut down on his or her usual activities for one whole day. Restricted activities by this definition do not require complete inactivity.

A person using the National Safety Council's definition could have different injury totals than a person using the definition given by the National Health Survey. This points out the need to define terms and to be sure which definition you are using at any given time. For our purposes, the terms used are always those defined by the National Safety Council.

death rates

Most death rates are expressed numerically on a "per year" basis in relationship to a unit of 100,000 people out of the entire population. For example, a "raw" death rate of 954 means that 954 people of all ages died from all causes per 100,000 people in the entire population within a given year. However "raw" this figure is, it does have some meaning. For instance, if you found that the birth rate in the United States was 4,000 per 100,000 of the population, you could easily determine that we were experiencing a growth rate in population—4,000 births versus 954 deaths per 100,000 population. If such were the case, this growth rate could be used in determining the number of schools or housing units required to meet future needs.

"Refined" death rates are more specific, providing more in-depth analysis for safety workers and people in the public health field. A refined death rate refers only to deaths from a specific cause. For example, a refined death rate of 58 from accidents simply means that 58 people per 100,000 population of all age groups died within one year from accidents. However, as pointed out in Chapter 1, more thorough analysis shows that in the age group 1–38, accidents are the leading killer. This puts an entirely different light on the situation. As one goes deeper into statistical analysis of accident data, additional findings may necessitate changes in the original interpretations of the data. Clearly, one must be careful not to base conclusions on insufficient evidence or inadequate analysis of the evidence.

injury rates

Industry separates injury rates into two categories—frequency and severity rates. Frequency rates refer to the "occurrence" of disabling injuries and are defined as the number of disabling injuries per 1,000,000 man-hours of exposure; the number of man-hours worked being the total number of man-hours worked in a given plant or department during a specified period of time. The computation is made as follows:

$$\text{Frequency rate} = \frac{\text{The number of disabling injuries} \times 1{,}000{,}000}{\text{Number of man-hours worked during the period}}$$

Since frequency rates take into account only occurrence and not severity, a severity rate must be calculated. The severity rate is the total days charged for work injuries per 1,000,000 man-hour exposure. The days charged include actual calendar days of disability for temporary total-disabling injuries. An example of a temporary total disability is a broken leg. An amputated leg would be a permanent disability. A fixed rate of 6,000 days is charged for death or permanent disability. Permanent partial disabilities are charged proportionately fewer days. The calculation of the severity rate is as follows:

$$\text{Severity rate} = \frac{\text{Number of days charged} \times 1{,}000{,}000}{\text{Number of man-hours worked during the period}}$$

Frequency and severity rates are most useful when they are calculated for several successive periods and then compared to see if an upward or downward trend is developing. Such a trend would be a good indicator of the effectiveness of safety measures and safety programs in a given industry. There are other indexes also used in industry for evaluation purposes, such as critical incidence and measurements of near misses; information on them can be found in industrial safety manuals.

CLASSIFICATION OF ACCIDENTAL
DEATHS AND INJURIES

The method of classifying accidental deaths and injuries depends on the intended use of the data and the amount of detail needed. For instance, the following classification is accidental death and disabling injuries by "class." Using this very general classification, the 1972 accidental death and injury picture appears as shown in Table 2-1.

Table 2-1. Principal classes of accidents, 1972.

	Deaths	Change from 1971	Disabling Injuries
Motor-Vehicle	**56,600**	**+3%**	**2,100,000**
Public non-work	52,400		2,000,000
Work	4,000		100,000
Home	200		10,000
Work	**14,100**	**−1%**	**2,400,000**
Non-motor-vehicle	10,100		2,300,000
Motor-vehicle	4,000		100,000
Home	**27,000**	**−2%**	**4,200,000**
Non-motor-vehicle	26,800		4,200,000
Motor-vehicle	200		10,000
Public	**23,500**	**+4%**	**2,900,000**

Reproduced from Accident Facts 1973 Edition, *p. 3, courtesy of the National Safety Council.*

When presenting such material, any unusual factors involved in the classification method should be pointed out to eliminate confusion and possible error in analysis. For example, it should be noted in this classification by principal classes that the deaths and injuries shown for the four separate classes of accidents total more than the national figures of 11,500,000 disabling injuries and 117,000 accidental deaths in 1972. That is because some deaths and injuries are included in more than one classification. For instance, 4,000 work deaths involved motor vehicles and are in both the work and motor vehicle classifications. Also 200 motor vehicle deaths occurred on home premises and are in both the home and motor vehicle classifications. The total of such duplication amounted to about 4,200 deaths and more than 100,000 disabling injuries.[2] This kind of explanation is the proper way to resent a set of accident statistics.

Despite its general nature, a classification of this type does have considerable value. For example, an investigator can readily see where most of the accidental deaths are occurring, and he can use this information to decide whether further and more detailed analysis is needed. If he wished to assign priorities to prevent such deaths, using this classification he might give primary emphasis to motor vehicle and home accidents in that order. However, extreme care should be taken with such general methods; a more detailed analysis or classification might result in assigning other priorities.

A more specific method classifies accidental deaths, injuries, and property damage by "accident type." This method describes the occurrence leading up to injury, death, or property damage. Deaths might be classified according to accident type by age groups, giving specific death rates while excluding other factors. In the following example, the classification includes accidental death by age for 1972 and excludes injuries and property damage losses.

This accident type classification method allows a much more specific analysis than does grouping by class. The addition of age groups adds further opportunity for detailed analysis. For example, in the 65 and older age groups, falls show up as an important cause of accidental death. You will also note an accompanying explanation indicating what deaths are included and excluded from each category. This is another example of the proper way to present accident data.

The classification by accident type shown in Figure 2-1 (pp. 18–19) gives a composite picture of the overall accidental death situation occurring in this country. Many priority decisions could be made from this type of accident grouping. Motor vehicle accidental deaths stand out. More in-depth analysis of motor vehicle crashes would reveal much other valuable information, such as the importance of alcohol as an aggravating factor. This information is obtained by classifying motor vehicle accidents according to cause (as will be shown in Chapter 4 on Traffic Safety).

The investigator can further refine the accident type approach by including sex and age with type, and can find other useful information. For example, Table 2-2 shows that in all age groups, except 75 and over,

2 National Safety Council, *Accident Facts 1973*, p. 3.

males have a consistently higher accidental death pattern than females. This could be significant in education and training programs for the prevention of accidents. (Again, caution must always be the rule when dealing with these types of statistics.)

Table 2-2. Accidental deaths by age, sex, and type.

Age and Sex	ALL TYPES	Motor-Vehicle	Falls	Drown-ing†	Fires, Burns*	Ingest. of Food, Object	Fire-arms	Poison (solid, liquid)	Poison by Gas	% Male All Types
All Ages......	116,385	55,791	17,827	7,699	7,163	3,712	2,309	2,967	1,549	69%
Under 5..........	6,973	2,077	325	800	1,012	1,012	80	245	45	58%
5 to 14..........	8,186	4,045	184	1,560	655	141	375	55	69	69%
15 to 24..........	24,668	17,443	389	2,190	396	256	777	676	405	80%
25 to 34..........	12,964	7,894	420	830	419	211	315	486	214	81%
35 to 44..........	11,446	5,974	742	710	636	295	253	415	238	76%
45 to 54..........	12,304	5,850	1,141	650	900	419	226	392	212	74%
55 to 64..........	11,888	5,162	1,766	480	1,053	415	170	342	188	71%
65 to 74..........	10,643	4,210	2,635	300	898	425	77	221	92	62%
75 & over.........	17,225	3,117	10,221	160	1,182	537	36	133	86	46%
Age unknown.....	88	19	4	19	12	1	0	2	0	76%
Sex										
Male..............	80,706	40,213	8,983	6,526	4,265	2,262	2,004	1,895	1,149	
Female...........	35,679	15,578	8,844	1,173	2,898	1,450	305	1,072	400	
Per cent male.....	69%	72%	50%	85%	60%	61%	87%	64%	74%	

Data are for 1969, latest official figures.

Reproduced from Accident Facts 1973 Edition, p. 14, courtesy of the National Safety Council.

Further refinements can include such factors as time of day, day of the week, month of the year, season of the year, weather conditions, and many others.

TRENDS IN ACCIDENT RATES

Between 1912 and 1972 accidental deaths were reduced 32 percent, from 82 to 56 per 100,000 population. The reduction in the overall rate during a period when the nation's population doubled meant that 1,550,000 fewer people were killed accidentally than would have been killed if the rate had not been reduced.[3] This is a significant accomplishment in the reduction of accidental death "rates."

As shown in Figure 2-2 (p. 20), trends are usually plotted on graphs that give a pictorial view of what is happening in a given situation.

Trends in accident death rates are subject to change because of improvements in some other area. Suppose that through increased enforcement procedures and better education techniques, we were nearly able to eliminate the alcohol factor in motor vehicle crashes. Theoreti-

[3] National Safety Council, Accident Facts 1973, p. 10.

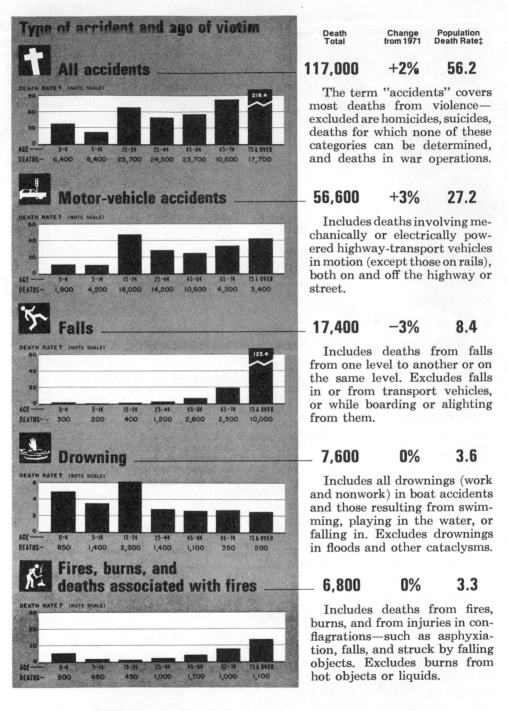

Type of accident and age of victim	Death Total	Change from 1971	Population Death Rate‡

✝ All accidents

117,000 +2% 56.2

DEATH RATE† (NOTE SCALE)

AGE—	0-4	5-14	15-24	25-44	45-64	65-74	75 & OVER
DEATHS—	6,400	8,400	25,700	24,500	23,700	10,600	17,700

218.4

The term "accidents" covers most deaths from violence— excluded are homicides, suicides, deaths for which none of these categories can be determined, and deaths in war operations.

Motor-vehicle accidents

56,600 +3% 27.2

DEATH RATE† (NOTE SCALE)

AGE—	0-4	5-14	15-24	25-44	45-64	65-74	75 & OVER
DEATHS—	1,900	4,200	18,000	14,200	10,600	4,300	3,400

Includes deaths involving mechanically or electrically powered highway-transport vehicles in motion (except those on rails), both on and off the highway or street.

Falls

17,400 −3% 8.4

DEATH RATE† (NOTE SCALE)

AGE—	0-4	5-14	15-24	25-44	45-64	65-74	75 & OVER
DEATHS—	300	200	400	1,200	2,800	2,500	10,000

123.4

Includes deaths from falls from one level to another or on the same level. Excludes falls in or from transport vehicles, or while boarding or alighting from them.

Drowning

7,600 0% 3.6

DEATH RATE† (NOTE SCALE)

AGE—	0-4	5-14	15-24	25-44	45-64	65-74	75 & OVER
DEATHS—	850	1,400	2,300	1,400	1,100	350	200

Includes all drownings (work and nonwork) in boat accidents and those resulting from swimming, playing in the water, or falling in. Excludes drownings in floods and other cataclysms.

Fires, burns, and deaths associated with fires

6,800 0% 3.3

DEATH RATE† (NOTE SCALE)

AGE—	0-4	5-14	15-24	25-44	45-64	65-74	75 & OVER
DEATHS—	900	650	450	1,000	1,700	1,000	1,100

Includes deaths from fires, burns, and from injuries in conflagrations—such as asphyxiation, falls, and struck by falling objects. Excludes burns from hot objects or liquids.

Figure 2-1. How people died accidentally in 1972. Reproduced from Accident Facts 1973 Edition, pp. 6–7, courtesy of the National Safety Council.

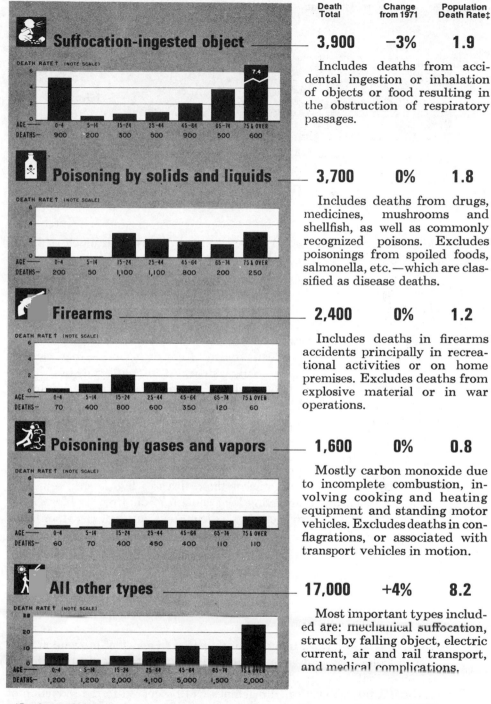

	Death Total	Change from 1971	Population Death Rate‡
Suffocation-ingested object	**3,900**	**−3%**	**1.9**

Includes deaths from accidental ingestion or inhalation of objects or food resulting in the obstruction of respiratory passages.

DEATH RATE† (NOTE SCALE)

AGE	0-4	5-14	15-24	25-44	45-64	65-74	75 & OVER
DEATHS	900	200	300	500	900	500	600

	Death Total	Change from 1971	Population Death Rate‡
Poisoning by solids and liquids	**3,700**	**0%**	**1.8**

Includes deaths from drugs, medicines, mushrooms and shellfish, as well as commonly recognized poisons. Excludes poisonings from spoiled foods, salmonella, etc.—which are classified as disease deaths.

DEATH RATE† (NOTE SCALE)

AGE	0-4	5-14	15-24	25-44	45-64	65-74	75 & OVER
DEATHS	200	50	1,100	1,100	800	200	250

	Death Total	Change from 1971	Population Death Rate‡
Firearms	**2,400**	**0%**	**1.2**

Includes deaths in firearms accidents principally in recreational activities or on home premises. Excludes deaths from explosive material or in war operations.

DEATH RATE† (NOTE SCALE)

AGE	0-4	5-14	15-24	25-44	45-64	65-74	75 & OVER
DEATHS	70	400	800	600	350	120	60

	Death Total	Change from 1971	Population Death Rate‡
Poisoning by gases and vapors	**1,600**	**0%**	**0.8**

Mostly carbon monoxide due to incomplete combustion, involving cooking and heating equipment and standing motor vehicles. Excludes deaths in conflagrations, or associated with transport vehicles in motion.

DEATH RATE† (NOTE SCALE)

AGE	0-4	5-14	15-24	25-44	45-64	65-74	75 & OVER
DEATHS	60	70	400	450	400	110	110

	Death Total	Change from 1971	Population Death Rate‡
All other types	**17,000**	**+4%**	**8.2**

Most important types included are: mechanical suffocation, struck by falling object, electric current, air and rail transport, and medical complications.

DEATH RATE† (NOTE SCALE)

AGE	0-4	5-14	15-24	25-44	45-64	65-74	75 & OVER
DEATHS	1,200	1,200	2,000	4,100	5,000	1,500	2,000

†Deaths per 100,000 population in each age group.　　　　‡Deaths per 100,000 population.

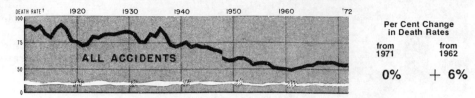

†Deaths per 100,000 population, adjusted to 1940 age distribution.

Figure 2-2. Trends in accidental death rates. Reproduced from Accident Facts 1973 Edition, *p. 10, courtesy of the National Safety Council.*

cally this could reduce motor vehicle related deaths by as much as 28,000 people per year. That fact would eventually show up as a very dramatic decrease in the trends in motor vehicle related accidental deaths. Over a period of ten years it could result in saving an estimated 280,000 lives. However, these same 280,000 people would die sometime; therefore, they would eventually appear in some other death statistic, either in diseases or accidents. Although some of them undoubtedly would still show up in a motor vehicle related death statistic from causes other than alcohol, a large number, for example, might show up in death statistics due to falls in the home. If enough of them did so, it could have a dramatic effect on trends in death rates due to falls in the home.

That is perhaps an oversimplified example, but it demonstrates how correcting one situation may shift emphasis to another. This phenomenon has occurred at times in medicine as the result of eliminating many diseases, such as smallpox, scarlet fever, or polio. Many of the people who might have died from one of those diseases live longer, some dying in accidents and many living long enough to die from problems associated with old age. Advances in medicine and accident reduction have extensive public health implications, such as increasing the average length of life in this country and inflating other cause-of-death statistics.

USING ACCIDENT DATA FOR RESEARCH PURPOSES

Accident research has a tremendous potential in accident prevention. Advanced technology and engineering will add many safety features to the machines that man operates in our complex society. Many of the features on these future sophisticated machines will be geared to the reduction of human error, which is responsible for approximately 80 percent of all accidents. However, we must also find ways of teaching people to do a better job of evaluating the hazards involved in the interaction process of man, machines, and environment. People must then be educated to exert better control over these hazards or react to them more effectively, especially under stress situations.

Significant gains in accident prevention can come from research into human behavior as it relates to accidents. As we have said, using accident data for any purpose requires certain precautions, and using it for research is no exception. These are some suggested precautions for using accident data for research purposes:

1. Define your terms well and limit your study carefully.
2. Obtain an adequate sample—there is safety in numbers.
3. Use adequate control groups and give special consideration to exposure. Check for stability of the individuals and be sure your groups are homogeneous.
4. Use both clinical and statistical approaches if necessary.
5. Be careful of men versus women studies.
6. Be careful of applying abstract psychological theories to statistical evidence. (This pitfall is discussed in Chapter 3.)
7. Examine carefully all reasonable alternative explanations.
8. Review previous similar studies and communicate directly with the researcher to gain the benefit of his experience.

SUMMARY

Valid accident data in sufficient quantity is a prerequisite to both originating and sustaining viable accident prevention programs. It is useful in determining priorities and establishing meaningful goals. Since lack of data retards our efforts in most areas of accident prevention, we must improve our present accident reporting systems.

Safety workers also should improve their own academic backgrounds, when needed, to insure more valid findings and avoid such common traps as basing conclusions on insufficient or erroneous data.

Accident data should be collected on a very systematic basis, completely analyzed, revalidated, applied in accident programs, reevaluated, and then reapplied. This type of approach will lay the groundwork for more efficient safety programs.

SUGGESTED STUDENT ACTIVITIES

1. Analyze a trend in a selected accident type and try to explain why the trend is acting in the manner you detect.

2. Design a proposed research study following the suggested guidelines for using accident data for research purposes.

3. Analyze the data in the various types of accidental deaths and assign priorities for accident prevention purposes.

4. Write a term paper on the common pitfalls in using accident data.

5. Make an analysis of motor vehicle accidents by time of day, month of year, and day of week. Make graphs to illustrate your analysis.

6. Select two different ways of analyzing motor vehicle death rates and discuss the weaknesses of each analysis.

7. Write a paper on the applicability of frequency rates versus severity rates.

8. Write a paper on accidents as a public health problem.

9. Find five ways to classify occupational accidents.

BIBLIOGRAPHY

NATIONAL SAFETY COUNCIL. *Accident Facts 1973 Edition.* Chicago, 1973.

3

understanding the causes of accidents

If accidents are to approach minimal levels, we must increase our understanding of their basic or root causes. Once these causes are more thoroughly understood, we can develop better education programs in accident prevention, and through technology, we can develop more efficient environmental controls and safer machinery.

CAUSES OF ACCIDENTS AS THEY RELATE TO LARGE HETEROGENEOUS GROUPS

When studying accidents, it is useful to consider the "causes" as they relate to large heterogeneous groups. An excellent example of this type of classification is given by A. E. Florio and G. T. Stafford. They classify accident causes into five general areas:

1. Inadequate knowledge.
2. Insufficient skill.
3. Environmental hazards.
4. Improper habits and attitudes.
5. Unsafe behavior.[1]

[1] A. E. Florio and G. T. Stafford, *Safety Education,* 3rd ed. (New York: McGraw-Hill, Inc., 1969), pp. 13–14.

inadequate knowledge

Knowledge is the foundation for understanding and the spring-board for the development of desirable attitudes toward safe behavior. Ideally every individual should learn and appreciate safety rules; unfortunately this is not always the case. The dramatic reduction in industrial accidents in recent years is the direct result of safety programs designed to educate the worker and, in turn, develop good habits and attitudes. We are realizing similar results with driver education programs. Every technological advance brings new hazards with which man must cope; thus education and the development of knowledge are a never-ending process. Adequate knowledge is vital if a person is to avoid hazardous situations and react properly when caught in such a situation. Also, proper knowledges enable the individual to recognize and evaluate dangerous situations.

insufficient skill

Attempting to perform tasks beyond one's ability level creates high-risk situations; thus skill level is an important determinant in accident prevention. Skill level is important in every facet of life and should be given primary consideration when participating in any activity, be it sports, work, or whatever. Skills are affected by many things, such as strength, fatigue, attitudes, emotions, alcohol, vision, and others.

environmental hazards

It is unrealistic to think that we can create a perfectly safe environment. Despite our inability to control our environment completely, only a small percentage of accidents are strictly environmental in nature. Society must "engineer out" as many environmental hazards as possible. Our present technology is advanced to the point where many hazards have been removed or controlled. Our present and future space programs may bring many new technological advances in environmental control. For example, the program may eventually enable us to control or modify weather and make more accurate weather predictions. Advances in this area will undoubtedly have some effects on accidents.

improper habits and attitudes

Great strides in accident reduction can be made by improving habits and attitudes. Every fact we know about accidents leads to the conclusion that faulty habits and attitudes are the prime accident producers. Every safety worker should thoroughly understand the development of attitudes and their possible modifications.

unsafe behavior

Unsafe behavior is the end result of man's failure to develop proper habits, attitudes, and knowledge concerning safety. Safe behavior entails responding correctly under all circumstances, and avoiding, when possible, high-risk situations. There is no excuse for purposely engaging in unsafe behavior.

PROXIMATE AND CASUAL CAUSES OF ACCIDENTS

Safety professionals generally agree that accidents are the result of many proximate and casual factors. These factors, or variables, interact to create unsafe acts and unsafe conditions, or both, which can terminate in an accident causing injury, death, or property damage.

An unsafe act or condition alone, or in some combination, if occurring at the right time may create an accident. (See Figure 3-1.) Remember, as implied by our definition, very few accidents occur by chance alone. Most accidents are caused.

There are thousands of variables in our daily lives which, if present under the right conditions, can produce an unsafe act or an unsafe con-

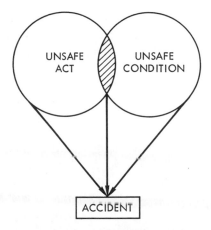

Figure 3-1. *Unsafe acts and unsafe conditions. Diagram courtesy of Jeanne V. Vitale.*

dition, or both. Figure 3-2 shows a few variables that could create an unsafe traffic "condition." Obviously, there are many more.

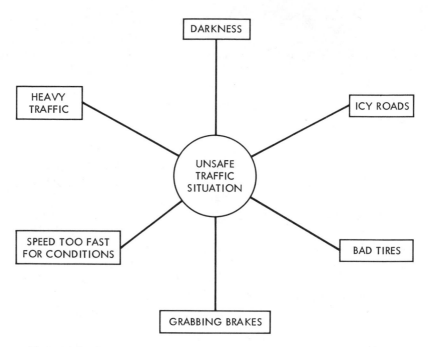

Figure 3-2. *Some contributing factors to an unsafe traffic condition.*

Figure 3-3 shows some of the many variables that, if present either alone or in some combination, could cause an unsafe "act."

Different variables, if present at the right time, under the right conditions, can produce a dangerous situation. Any one alone can do so. The more variables present, naturally the higher the risk. In other words, the more variables present, the greater the opportunity for the timing factor to operate. Timing is catalytic in a sense, enabling all the forces to interact in the "proper" order to cause an accident.

The variables, or contributing factors, in a given situation are relative. For example, the alcohol factor would be more significant in heavy traffic than in light traffic. Icy roads become more significant in heavy traffic than in light. The combination of icy roads, heavy traffic, and alcohol-involved drivers creates an even higher risk situation. For further aggravation, we can include an emotionally upset person. With this combination of high-risk factors, an accident would seem inevitable. The ability to prevent such an accident will depend on the following:

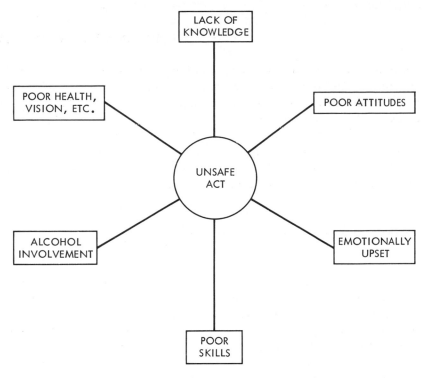

Figure 3-3. Some contributing factors to an unsafe act in traffic.

1. Proper recognition of the variables present.
2. Understanding the relative significance of the variables present—proper evaluation.
3. Removing the hazards if possible—not driving in this case.
4. Making the proper behavioral response in traffic. (Compensation —difficult to do under the circumstances.)

In reality, there is only one safe choice in such a situation. After recognizing the variables present and evaluating them, the driver should not drive. But will his or her judgment be impaired to the point where a wrong decision is made? Either the alcohol or emotional upset could precipitate a wrong decision. This identical situation will develop thousands of times during the next year. Many will not make a rational decision, and many will perish. Some will escape because, through luck or compensation, timing failed to establish the forces present in the order necessary to create an accident.

AN ACCIDENT IN A SYSTEM

Sometimes the sequence of events leading up to an accident is readily traceable, as in the following illustration. John, a normally stable individual, is having either conscious or subconscious job-related problems. He leaves for work on Monday morning, fifteen minutes behind his normal schedule. It is a clear day. He is driving on a narrow two-way street, with heavy rush-hour traffic. As he approaches point "A" he is caught behind a bus loading passengers, a fairly common occurrence. Oncoming traffic prevents his passing. The bus continues down the street,

A   B   C   D   E   F   G   H

stopping at every intersection to load more passengers. John's emotions begin to build up after he glances at his watch and notices that he is losing more and more time. His desire to reach the office on time is overpowering. Finally, at point "H" he sees a chance to pass the bus and decides to do so. His perception has been badly impaired by the emotional crisis. A head-on crash occurs. In making a close analysis of this situation, it could honestly be said that although the accident occurred at point "H," it actually started at point "A."

Preventing this accident would have required an interruption in the sequence of events leading up to the crash. There are many proximate and casual causes in this case. Obviously, John's emotional upset was the triggering factor. He should have evaluated the situation more closely, recognized his emotional stress and other dangerous variables, such as heavy traffic, and then taken compensating action.

Simply by retracing the events and variables present, John's particular motor vehicle accident can be explained. However, if we are to reduce similar accidents to an irreducible minimum, we must consider the whole system in which the accident occurred and not just the accident itself. There may have been many malfunctions in the system, which includes John, his car, and his environment, that contributed equally to the accident.

Where did the system fail? Why didn't John take special precautions during his emotional upset? This indicates a failure in our education process. Could the street have been made less dangerous through traffic engineering? For example, would the street have been safer and more efficient if it had been designated as "one way"? What could have been changed to keep the bus from blocking traffic at every intersection? Should the bus stop have been on the far side of the intersection? Were there any structural defects in the cars that impaired the drivers' vision or ability to control their vehicles?

Obviously we need to examine the entire system in which the accident occurred to determine all the proximate and casual causes. Such an analysis would undoubtedly turn up many heretofore unnoticed contributing causes in similar accidents. The more proximate and casual causes exposed, the greater the opportunity to determine the root causes of these accidents. Once root causes are fully determined, future accident probability in similar situations can be diminished. Such an analysis would provide the foundation for better education, better automotive engineering, and better environmental engineering. All parts of the system—man, his machines, and his environment—must interact together in a smooth and efficient manner to promote optimum safety.

SYSTEMS SAFETY ANALYSIS: A MODERN APPROACH TO SAFETY PROBLEMS

Note: This section is a reprint of an article by J. L. Recht, Assistant Director Statistics Division, National Safety Council, and is reprinted courtesy of the Council.[2]

We have all heard that this is the space age. But, except for following the exploits of the astronauts and looking at pictures of the moon and Mars, most of us have not felt the impact of the new technology which has made the space age a reality. This new technology has produced new hardware—rockets, missiles, and supersonic aircraft—but these products are only the tangible results of the new analytical methods and new theoretical concepts which form the core of our advancing technology.

For those of us in the safety field, this situation is likely to change rapidly. Concepts currently in use in the aerospace industries—which can be described by the phrase "systems safety analysis"—are beginning to have important ramifications in other industrial fields.

Systems safety analysis is not an ill-defined approach to safety or a phrase that masks the same old approaches—it is in fact a concept so well-developed in the industries closely involved with space programs that recent Department of Defense military specifications require the application of systems safety analytical techniques as part of contract terms, and it appears that such requirements could spread beyond the aerospace industry. Systems safety approaches are also being utilized to analyze product safety in a few private industrial establishments.

[2] J. L. Recht, *Systems Safety Analysis: A Modern Approach to Safety Problems*, special publication (Chicago: National Safety Council, n.d.), pp. 1–4.

In the years to come, safetymen will hear more and more about systems safety—and most of what they hear will be couched in the special vocabulary that has developed among aerospace systems safety engineers.

Safetymen will not only hear about these techniques, they will have to understand them, for many will be called on to find ways of implementing them. And although complete implementation of systems safety analysis involves specially-trained engineers and rather sophisticated mathematical manipulations, safetymen will find that knowledge of the most rudimentary facets of these techniques can be of direct benefit in helping codify and direct their accident prevention programs.

Why systems safety?

The history of systems safety analysis really began in the aerospace industry. It was the result of the extremely high reliability and safety specifications demanded by the space and military requirements and the fact that the time-honored production sequence was no longer practical.

Until recently, when a new aircraft was developed, it was first designed, then an experimental model was built, and finally it was test-flown to determine its capabilities and flaws; the information obtained indicated the necessary design changes and the cycle was repeated until the performance specifications were met. Today's aircraft and missiles are so complex and costly and the specifications are set so high that this procedure had to be changed. Moreover, missile flight tests involve loss of the model with only limited telemetry data obtained. Today the "bugs" must be found and corrected as far as possible in the design stage using analytical techniques.

The result is the development of the systems approach to safety. The aircraft or missile is examined from this point of view and the effects of any failures or malfunctions on the operation of the aircraft are evaluated to determine the principal design defects which need to be fixed. For these complex systems, sophisticated analytical methods have been developed using high-speed computers. Thus the test pilot has been replaced by a systems safety engineer and a computer. The objective, "First time safe," is quite different from the objective of investigating accidents and preventing recurrences.

For simpler systems merely having an understanding of the systems approach can have great benefits. This article is an effort to introduce and *define* systems terminology. . . .

What is a system?

To understand the systems approach we should first have a clear picture of what a system is. Definitions tend to be restricting, but one which might serve our purposes is the following:

A system is an orderly arrangement of components which are interrelated and which act and interact to perform some task or function in a particular environment.

The main points to keep in mind are that a system is defined in terms of a task or function (it is task-oriented), and that the components of a system are interrelated, that is, each part affects the others.

The task or function which a system performs may be simple or complex. Sometimes it is convenient to break up a complex task into simpler tasks and consider subsystems of the larger system. Subsystems consist of part of the components of the over-all system and perform a portion of the over-all task.

System components

The components of a system can cover a wide range including machines, tools, material (i.e. hardware, chemicals, etc.), environmental factors, people, documents (such as operating instructions, training manuals, or computer programs), and so on. As parts of a system, the components usually complement each other but it is essential to recognize that a failure or malfunction of any component can affect the other components and thus degrade the performance of the task.

The environment is an important consideration in a system since most systems will perform their task properly only under a given set of conditions. A component that works well at normal temperatures may be placed in a system near another component that generates high heat and thus the first component will not function properly. The environment in which the components operate must always, therefore, be considered as a part of a system and be included in any examination of a system.

A sample system

An automatic gas hot-water heater is a good example to use in illustrating the elements of a system. The task of the system is to provide hot water in our house at all times. In order to perform this task a system is used whose components consist of a water tank, a gas heater, a temperature measuring and comparing device to regulate the system, a controller (actuated by the temperature measuring device) to turn a valve, a gas valve to control the flow of the gas, a pressure relief value (to permit excess pressure to escape if the gas heater fails to shut off), a cold water intake pipe, a hot water pipe leading to the faucets, and an exhaust pipe for the flue gases from the gas heater.

From the view of task performance, we can examine the system to see in what ways failure or malfunction of the components can stop delivery of hot water when we want it, or, more importantly, when the system might get out of control and the tank rupture or gas escape. The interrelations of the components are apparent to anyone familiar with the operation of such a heater and we can trace through the system the effects of any component breakdown.

Another example which is not completely mechanical is the system for waking you up in the morning. The task is waking you at the desired time. The system components consist of an alarm clock, you, and the environment. The clock (which here is a subsystem) must be in good working condition to perform the task, but this is not sufficient. The clock must be wound, the time set correctly, and the alarm button pulled—you perform these operations.

In addition, if the clock is kept under conditions of abnormal heat, moisture, dust, and so on, it will eventually fail to function as it should and the alarm system will not perform its task.

Again it is relatively easy to see the interrelationships of the components and the effects of any malfunction on task performance.

Analyzing systems

Having established the concept of a system, the next step is the analysis of systems—especially complex systems such as aircraft, communications networks, or production lines. It is in this area—the analysis of complex systems—that great progress has been made in recent years in the aerospace industry which holds great promise for application throughout industry.

It is not possible in an introductory article to describe in detail each of the analytical methods which have been developed. However, it might be helpful to indicate briefly the main techniques in order to clarify the nature of the systems approach to safety.

No matter which method of analysis is used, it is important to have a model of the system. Most models take the form of a diagram showing *all* the components. This makes it easier to grasp the interrelationships and simplifies tracing the effects of malfunctions.

Methods of analysis

There are four principal methods of analysis: failure mode and effect, fault tree, THERP, and cost-effectiveness. Each has a number of variations and more than one may be combined in a single analysis.

Failure mode and effect

In the failure mode and effect method, failure or malfunction of each component is considered including the mode of failure (such as, switch jammed "on"), the effects of the failure are traced through the system, and the ultimate effect on the task performance is evaluated. Failure mode and effect analysis is straightforward assuming that the analyst is thoroughly informed about the system. One drawback of this method, however, is that it considers only one failure at a time and thus some possibilities may be overlooked.

Fault tree

In the fault tree method an undesired event is selected and all the possible happenings that can contribute to the event are diagrammed in the form of a tree. The branches of the tree are continued until independent events are reached. Probabilities are determined for the independent events and after simplifying the tree, both the probability of the undesired event and the most likely chain of events leading up to it can be computed.

This is a very powerful analysis technique but has the drawback of requiring a fairly heavy mathematical background and a good computer to obtain the maximum benefits of the method. Boeing Company has refined the fault tree method to a high degree and has found it practical for analyzing aerospace products.

THERP

THERP, technique for human error prediction, developed by Sandia Corporation, provides a means for quantitatively evaluating the contribution of human error to the degradation of product quality. It can be used for human components in systems and thus can be combined either with the failure mode and effect or the fault tree methods.

Cost effectiveness

In the cost effectiveness method, the cost of system changes made to increase safety are compared with either the decreased costs of fewer serious failures, or with the increased effectiveness of the system to perform its task, to determine the relative value of these changes. Ultimately all system changes have to be costed, but this method makes such cost comparisons explicit. Moreover, cost-effectiveness is frequently used to help make decisions concerning the choice of one of several systems which can perform the same task.

In all of these analytical methods the main point is to measure quantitatively the effects of various failures within a system. In each case probability theory is an important element.

Zero defects programs

In the aerospace industry there are a number of programs called "zero defects" programs with such interesting names as: Pride, Aware, Esky, Project Sterling, and others. These are primarily quality control programs aimed at motivating greater attention to product quality. They are not systems safety analysis programs in the strict sense. Safety naturally should be improved but this is a secondary rather than a primary objective of these programs. ZD programs are a consequence of the extremely high specifications now set for aerospace products.

The industrial safety engineer might well ask what all this systems analysis has to do with him. The answer to that question, and the major point of this article, is that anyone can use and profit from the systems approach to safety. The systems notion helps to enlarge one's viewpoint. Becoming oriented in terms of task performance and being forced to visualize the interrelationships of all the components of a system helps to bring most accident possibilities into consideration automatically and in an orderly manner.

The systems approach to safety can help to change safety engineering from an art to a science by codifying much of our knowledge. It can change the application of safety from piece-meal problem solving (putting a pan under the leak) to a safely designed operation (avoiding the leak itself). We can apply the question "what can happen if this component fails" to the various elements of the systems and come up with adequate safety answers *before* the accident occurs instead of after the damage has been done.

A PSYCHOLOGICAL APPROACH TO ACCIDENT CAUSES

Statistical evidence over the past several years consistently points to the fact that approximately 20 percent of the people have most of the accidents, while the remaining 80 percent remain relatively free from accidents.[3] Another statistic generally accepted today is that approximately 80 percent of accidents are caused by human error.

[3] N. R. Lykes, *A Psychological Approach to Accidents* (New York: Vantage Press, Inc., 1954), pp. 10–11.

Such evidence immediately leads the investigator into the field of social psychology or human behavior. Literature on human behavior reveals much confusion concerning attitudes, emotions, and perceptions. Some of the confusion centers around the inability to measure these characteristics effectively. The confusion makes investigation difficult.

Accident investigation is further aggravated by another problem, as Bruce D. Greenshields points out. He says that since attitudes and emotions are not among the reported causes of accidents, there is no accurate information about their importance in the accident picture.[4]

Another stumbling block is the fact that any investigation of attitudes, emotions, and perceptions must inevitably give consideration to the central nervous system, another area not completely understood. However, even under such handicaps, we should work harder, cooperate more fully with all disciplines, and attempt to reach understanding heretofore beyond our grasp. This only supports the contention that accident investigation involves many disciplines, none of them mutually exclusive of each other. It seems obvious that those involved in accident investigation and prevention should have a solid background in human behavior, with knowledge and understanding of the central nervous system.

The field of human behavior is most complicated, but there is general agreement in at least some areas. Apparently there is a chainlike reaction involving attitudes, emotions, and perceptions. Attitudes, which are expressions of the total personality, determine how strongly we feel about something. They have a direct effect upon emotions, at times causing wild swings in emotional levels. Emotions, in turn, affect perception, or the way we see a given situation. Figure 3-4 diagrams how attitudes, emotions, and perceptions interact.

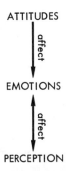

Figure 3-4. The interaction of attitudes, emotions, and perception.

[4] Bruce D. Greenshields, "Attitudes, Emotions, and Accidents," *Traffic Quarterly,* April 1959, p. 222.

Note that the arrow in the diagram runs both ways between emotions and perception. This is because perception, or the way we see something, can also affect emotions. For instance, witnessing a bad accident can be a traumatic experience, and can cause perceptual distortion, which results in several different and conflicting eyewitness accounts of the accident and the event in general.

attitudes

An attitude is defined by Robert M. Goldenson as "a response, favorable or unfavorable, to a person, group, idea or situation." [5]

Most psychologists think of attitudes as predispositions to act. James Deese says they are not actions themselves but are conditions within ourselves which cause us to react in certain ways.[6] In a statement relating to driving, C. T. Perrin says that proper attitudes toward safety make the behavior of people predictable, and undesirable attitudes cause unpredictable, erratic, and unsafe behavior in driving situations.[7]

Human behaviorists believe that attitudes arise from human needs, but are based on knowledge and experience. However, not all knowledge and experience contribute to desirable attitudes toward safe behavior. For example, a child may hear his parents or friends brag about "high-speed" exploits in an automobile, and may develop undesirable attitudes toward speed. He may hear his parents downgrade a law enforcement officer, and may develop poor attitudes toward the police and others engaged in law enforcement.

A person's behavior will generally be governed by the attitudes he has formed toward that class of experiences. Goldenson points out that attitudes are developed through experience and tend to resist change.[8] For example, a speed enthusiast would tend to resist a lesson on speed. A person who resents authority and restriction on his behavior might view traffic regulations as unnecessary. He might tend to disregard them when driving. On the other hand, a person who sees traffic regulations as a social regulation for his own protection would obey these laws and be a much safer driver.

Educators should take a lesson from this and develop specific strategies to insure that their teaching is positive and conducive to safe behavior; then go a step further and continuously reinforce this learning.

[5] Robert M. Goldenson, *The Encyclopedia of Human Behavior, Psychology, Psychiatry, and Mental Health* (Garden City, N.Y.: Doubleday & Company, Inc., 1970), 1:127.

[6] James Deese, *General Psychology* (Boston: Allyn & Bacon, Inc., 1967), p. 491.

[7] C. T. Perrin, "Our Failure to Apply Psychology to the Field of Driver Safety," *Traffic Digest and Review*, September 1960, p. 25.

[8] Goldenson, *Encyclopedia of Human Behavior*, 1:128.

Positive teaching with constant reinforcement for safe behavior is utilized in the nation's better flying schools. Every technique about flying is taught with safety in mind. For example, flying instructors start with "This is the safe way to enter the airplane." The phrase, "This is the safe way" prefaces the teaching of every new skill or knowledge related to flying. The end result is the accumulation of much desirable knowledge and many desirable habits and attitudes. This is manifested by a fine safety record in commercial aviation and a much better record in private aviation than is generally thought.

The effects of constant reinforcement cannot be over-stressed. A classic example is that of the Coca Cola Company. For years it installed signs at almost every possible location advertising Coke as "the pause that refreshes." Consequently, the name Coke is well ingrained in the public mind. How frequently do you hear someone say, "Let's stop and have (some other name brand of cola)"? If continual reinforcement was unimportant, large corporations would not spend endless sums of money on advertising. If we can control human behavior through this type of reinforcement, it stands to reason that the constant reinforcement of safety techniques can affect our behavior where personal safety is concerned.

modification of attitudes

Modifying undesirable attitudes toward safety is a very important part of accident prevention. Attitudes tend to resist change because they are self preservative in nature. The stronger the attitude, the harder it will be to change. For example, changing attitudes toward religion and politics can be very difficult.

Before we can effectively design strategies for modifying an attitude, we must know certain things about the attitude. We need to know about the knowledges and beliefs upon which it is based. What new information will have to be added 'to change it? For example, a thorough explanation of the effects of speed on "force of impact" might cause a person to change an undesirable attitude about speed.

We should also know what pleasures the person derives from maintaining an attitude. Does he get recognition from his peers because of it? If so, we need to find substitutes that would replace this desired recognition.

People with undesirable attitudes toward safety tend to resent authority. Since the teacher represents authority to these people, he or she must be extremely careful in attempting to modify undesirable attitudes. However, one of the better ways in which a skillful teacher can bring about a change in undesirable attitudes is through class discussion. By carefully guiding a discussion on speed, for example, the teacher may cause an individual's peers to express themselves openly in such a manner as to show that they do not respect those with undesirable attitudes about safe behavior. The effect on Johnny, the speed enthusiast, when he learns that the girls in his class do not like to ride with habitual speeders could be dramatic.

We must know how an attitude fits into the total personality of an individual. Then specific counter measures can be tailor-made to fit the situation. Although attitudes do resist change, the fact that they can be modified offers great hope to those working in accident prevention.

emotions

Emotion is defined by Goldenson in a general way as " 'stirred up' feeling, usually directed toward a specific person or event, and involving widespread visceral and skeletal changes." [9]

While others might describe emotion in such terms as hate, love, or anger, there is general agreement that emotions fluctuate and vary in intensity. They involve widespread visceral and skeletal changes. S. K. Fitch lists some of these as: [10]

1. Skin changes (galvanic skin response).
2. Pupillary response (pupils dilate during excitement).
3. Blood distribution (face flushes).
4. Heart and blood pressure increase.
5. Respiratory changes.
6. Salivary secretion.

Some of these changes can be detected by the naked eye, such as dilation of the pupils or flushing of the face. When emotions fluctuate, they create "moods," sometimes referred to as emotional states. Everyone's emotions fluctuate from day to day depending on the day's events. No one is absolutely free of stress or excitement. Most people tend to stay somewhat within a normal range unless something drastic happens, such as the death of a loved one. It is when people get too elated or too depressed that they apparently exceed their particular tolerance level. Therefore, people should automatically become more cautious during such periods. We should definitely orientate people to this phenomenon.

According to B. B. Hersey, in a study of more than 440 industrial accidents, approximately one half of them occurred when the workers were in a low emotional state. He also found that approximately 20 percent of the observed accidents happened when the workers were in an

[9] Goldenson, *Encyclopedia of Human Behavior,* 1:387.
[10] S. K. Fitch, *Insights into Human Behavior* (Boston: Hollbrook Press, 1970), pp. 131–33.

elated state. Hersey estimated that workers are in a low emotional state not more than 20 percent of the time, which would indicate that a worker is four times as likely to have an accident in a low emotional state as in a normal state.[11] Figure 3-5 illustrates how emotions vary in depth and intensity.

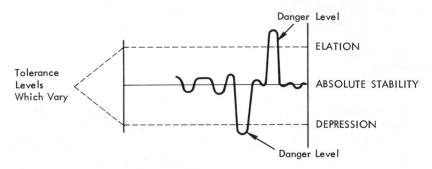

Figure 3-5. Human emotional tolerance levels.

Although this represents just one study, it reinforces our understanding of the effects of emotions on human behavior. The big problem is to find the critical level of emotional stress. Apparently it varies from person to person. We need extensive experimental data concerning tolerance limits of emotional stress and how they are affected by different stimuli.

perception

Perception is defined in Goldenson's *Encyclopedia of Human Behavior* as "The process of becoming aware of objects, qualities, or relations via the sense organs; includes such activities as observing, recognizing, discriminating and grasping meaning." [12]

The process of perception involves more than merely recognizing, but also includes organizing and interpreting data. The difference between perception and attention is that attention focuses in on a narrow range of stimuli while perception interprets the stimuli.

This process of interpretation determines our reaction—pleasant or unpleasant—to a particular stimulus. In avoidance of accidents, perception is of vital importance. In order to react correctly we must have proper interpretation.

[11] B. B. Hersey, "Emotional Factors in Accidents," *Personnel Journal*, vol. 16, 1937.

[12] Goldenson, *Encyclopedia of Human Behavior*, 2:936.

A person experiences perceptual distortion, causing misinterpretation under certain circumstances. Perceptual distortion, according to Goldenson, can occur from any of the following:

1. Drugs.
2. Severe mental disease.
3. Sensory deprivation.
4. Influence of the individual needs, values, and attitudes.[13]

All of these have a direct or indirect effect on emotions. Attitudes, emotions, and perceptions need continued research if we are to promote accident reduction. The development and modification of attitudes rate primary consideration in safety education.

ACCIDENT PRONENESS THEORIES

In 1919 Major Greenwood and Hilda M. Woods, two British researchers, reported that a relatively low percentage of workers they studied had a higher percentage of the accidents than would be expected by chance alone. This electrifying research in the history of accident prevention caused a proliferation of theories, generated much research, and created a lot of confusion, much of which still exists today.

This study was followed by Karl Marbe, a German psychologist, who showed through a series of studies from 1922 to 1926 that the individual who had one accident was more likely to have another than was the individual who never experienced an accident. This supports the general agreement that approximately 80 percent of accidents involve approximately 20 percent of people.

Many studies have been conducted to identify some psychological or personality trait associated with this statistical phenomenon. However, no one has been able to identify a trait that is common only to those people who have unduly high accident rates. This precludes accident prediction via a psychological testing device.

Possibly many people have tended to confuse accident repetitiveness with accident proneness. It is a well established fact that certain people at certain times are accident repeaters. A study of two groups, one accident repeaters and the other accident free, will show that the groups interchange to some extent in subsequent studies. This has led to the theory that if accident proneness does in fact exist, it is variable in nature.

[13] Goldenson, *Encyclopedia of Human Behavior*, 2:938–39.

Individual cases of accident proneness may exist, but a major portion of accident repetitiveness cannot be explained in this way.[14] The phenomenon of accident proneness has not been conclusively proven. It does, however, deserve further consideration.

Morris Schulzinger suggests a clinical approach: all people, including those who have had an accident, should be considered from the standpoint of their current state of health, emotional stability, family backgrounds, and other factors, plus their past history of behavior under stress.[15]

HEALTH AS AN ETIOLOGICAL FACTOR IN ACCIDENTS

Authorities generally agree that health is an extremely important factor in accident prevention. As it relates to etiology (the assignment of cause), health impairment makes one more susceptible to accidents. Employers in various industries, airlines for example, require vigorous physical examinations for their employees.

C. P. Yost says that factors causing accidents are either directly or indirectly related to health. The degree of fitness may in many cases determine whether or not an accident will occur. One study of industrial accidents found that the leading causes of accidents, regardless of sex, were visual and auditory defects, poor motor and reflex coordination, alcoholism, and fatigue. Factors such as menstruation, pregnancy, lactation, and menopause were leading causes of accidents among women.[16]

As far back as 1927, a study by C. S. Slocombe and W. F. Bingham showed that the physical condition of street car and motor bus operators, as measured by blood pressure, was a factor in safe performance.[17]

There is no question about the importance of vision in accident prevention. Approximately 90 percent of our driving decisions depend on vision. People with poor depth perception and visual acuity must compensate for the deficiency when driving.

Factors such as lack of sleep and rest, which cause excessive fatigue,

[14] William Haddon, Jr., Edward A. Suchman, and David Klein, *Accident Research, Methods and Approaches,* Association for the Aid of Crippled Children (New York: Harper & Row, 1964), p. 417.

[15] Morris Schulzinger, "The Accident Syndrome," *National Safety Congress Transactions* 6 (1961):66.

[16] C. P. Yost, "The Values of Total Fitness in Preventing Accidents," *National Safety Council Transactions* 23 (1961):21.

[17] C. S. Slocombe and W. F. Bingham, "Men Who Have Accidents," *Personnel Journal* 6 (1927):251–57.

are possible accident producers. Conditions such as epilepsy or diabetes, which can produce seizures, have accident-producing potential. For example, the epileptic may suffer a seizure while taking a shower and become scalded if he falls against the hot water valve, or he may suffer a seizure while driving and crash. In fact, the first responsibility in administering first aid to epileptics is to get them into a position where they can do no harm to themselves.

Any of the manifestations of poor circulation, such as numbness, dizziness, fatigue, general weakness, and heart failure, can cause an accident. Dizziness is a leading cause of falls, especially among older people.

Many problems associated with old age have accident implications —brittle bones for example. An older person slips, causing a sudden and unexpected shift of weight to the opposite foot. The shift causes a brittle bone to break, with a resulting fall. In many such cases the fall is diagnosed as the cause of the break, instead of the brittle bone (a health factor) causing the break, with the ensuing fall.

Alcoholism is rated by some as the number one health problem in this country. There is ample evidence of its effects on traffic accidents, as well as other types. Drug abuse is another cause of serious accidents. Any drug that can alter reaction time, reflexes, or mental conditions must be considered capable of producing high-risk situations.

Auditory defects prevent people from hearing possible warnings that could prevent an accident. Balance is also affected by health defects or conditions in the middle ear.

Neurological defects and diseases affecting the central and autonomic nervous system create health conditions that make a person more susceptible to accidents. Nutritional deficiencies, with their manifestations in poor vision or muscular weakness, are potential accident producers.

A healthy person is a safer person: As we have said, everyone has the responsibility to maintain good health as an accident-prevention measure. For remedial purposes, accident reporting forms should give more attention to health factors as possible proximate and casual causes of accidents.

PERSONAL ACCIDENT POTENTIAL

Every individual has some potential for becoming involved in an accident, since there is an element of risk in all of our activities. Even in sleep, for example, there is the danger of fire, or the remote possibility of a car or airplane roaring into the bedroom. Activities carry with them varying degrees of accident potential. Much of the potential for an accident in different activities depends on the individual. His health, skill level, emotional tolerance limits, or exposure rates are important personal variables.

For large groups of people, we can predict with some accuracy that accidents will occur. For example, the National Safety Council forecasts with grim success the number of people who will die in traffic accidents during holiday periods. However, it is impossible to predict when a given person will have an accident. In fact, we cannot say with accuracy that a given person, at a given time, is even accident susceptible. Remember, the accident occurs only if the certain variables are present under the right conditions at the right time. We cannot predict when that situation will develop. We do know, however, that the more possible accident-triggering variables present, the better the chances for an accident to occur.

If for no other reason than to create a higher level of safety awareness, it is useful to make self-evaluations to determine strengths and weaknesses that might make one more or less accident prone. You can rate yourself in the diagrams that follow. After rating yourself, let others rate you; then ask yourself the following questions. What are my strengths and weaknesses? Do I need to compensate for certain factors under certain circumstances?

A low reading on any one of these scales alone does not necessarily mean that you have high accident potential, but it does indicate a condition of which you should be aware. A low rating across the board would be a cause for high concern. Recognize and evaluate, then compensate or remove the hazards involved if possible. You will be a safer and happier person.

Figure 3-6. How do you rate yourself?

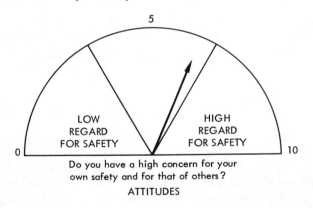

ATTITUDES

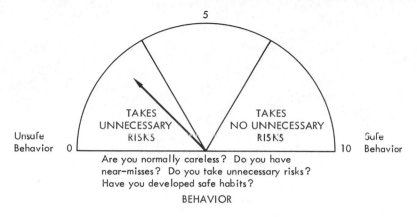

5

Unsafe
Behavior   0

TAKES
UNNECESSARY
RISKS

TAKES
NO UNNECESSARY
RISKS

10   Safe
Behavior

Are you normally careless? Do you have
near-misses? Do you take unnecessary risks?
Have you developed safe habits?

BEHAVIOR

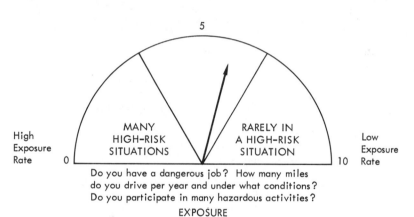

5

High
Exposure
Rate   0

MANY
HIGH-RISK
SITUATIONS

RARELY IN
A HIGH-RISK
SITUATION

10   Low
Exposure
Rate

Do you have a dangerous job? How many miles
do you drive per year and under what conditions?
Do you participate in many hazardous activities?

EXPOSURE

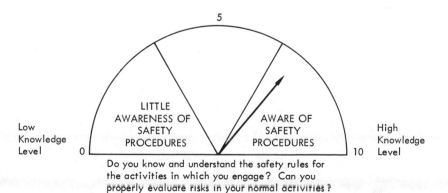

5

Low
Knowledge
Level   0

LITTLE
AWARENESS OF
SAFETY
PROCEDURES

AWARE OF
SAFETY
PROCEDURES

10   High
Knowledge
Level

Do you know and understand the safety rules for
the activities in which you engage? Can you
properly evaluate risks in your normal activities?

KNOWLEDGE

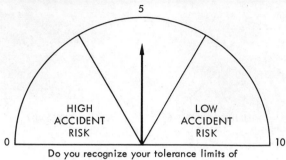

Do you recognize your tolerance limits of
emotional fluctuation? Do you have
violent emotional swings?

MENTAL STABILITY

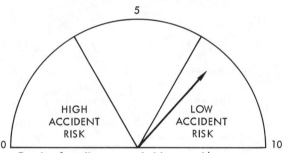

Freedom from disease, good vision, good heart, etc.
Do you have any health defects that could possibly
trigger an accident?

PHYSICAL HEALTH

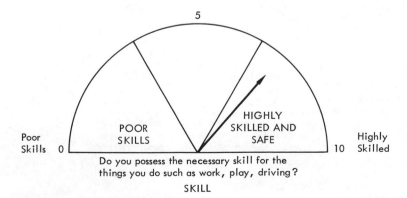

Do you possess the necessary skill for the
things you do such as work, play, driving?

SKILL

SUMMARY

Approximately 115,000 accidental deaths per year, accompanied by millions of disabling injuries, represent a malignancy in our society. These accidents result from many proximate and casual causes, making the field of accident investigation and prevention very complex. In order to make significant progress in accident reduction, we must increase our present knowledge relating to accident causes, giving consideration to the entire system in which the accident occurred and not just the accident itself.

Attitudes, emotions, and perceptions provide the biggest area for improvement in accident prevention. Human error resulting primarily from faulty habits and attitudes apparently is the prime producer of accidents. Our research efforts must be stepped up in this area. We need research into the possible ways of effectively creating and modifying attitudes and human behavior.

Our teaching methods must be positive in nature. Constant reinforcement of safety knowledges and practices should be a standard procedure.

SUGGESTED STUDENT ACTIVITIES

1. Prepare a self-evaluation scale of your own habits, attitudes, exposure, and other factors.
2. Design a paper on the strategy for changing an attitude.
3. Visit an industry or police department and make an anatomical study of an actual accident. (See Figure 5-3, "The anatomy of a fall in the home.")
4. Prepare a graph showing the relationship between diseases and accidents.
5. Select an occupation and prepare a list of the primary health prerequisites for that job.
6. Write a paper on the personality characteristics of a safe person.
7. Review three research papers and compare the common personality characteristics, if any, of an accident repeater.

BIBLIOGRAPHY

DEESE, JAMES. *General Psychology.* Boston: Allyn & Bacon, Inc., 1967.

FITCH, S. K. *Insights into Human Behavior.* Boston: Hollbrook Press, 1970.

FLORIO, A. E., and STAFFORD, G. T. *Safety Education.* 3rd ed. New York: McGraw-Hill, Inc., 1969.

GOLDENSON, ROBERT M. *The Encyclopedia of Human Behavior, Psychology, Psychiatry, and Mental Health.* Vols. 1 & 2. Garden City, N. Y.: Doubleday & Company, Inc., 1970.

GREENSHIELDS, BRUCE D. "Attitudes, Emotions, and Accidents." *Traffic Quarterly,* April 1959, p. 222.

HADDON, WILLIAM, JR.; SUCHMAN, EDWARD; and KLEIN, DAVID. *Accident Research, Methods and Approaches.* Association for the Aid of Crippled Children. New York: Harper & Row, 1964.

HERSEY, B. B. "Emotional Factors in Accidents." *Personnel Journal* 16 (1937).

LYKES, N. R. *A Psychological Approach to Accidents.* New York: Vantage Press, Inc., 1954.

PERRIN, C. T. "Our Failure to Apply Psychology in the Field of Driver Safety." *Traffic Digest and Review,* September 1960, p. 25.

RECHT, J. L. *Systems Safety Analysis: A Modern Approach to Safety Problems.* Special publication. Chicago: National Safety Council, n.d.

SCHULZINGER, MORRIS. "The Accident Syndrome." *National Safety Congress Transactions* 6 (1961): 66.

SLOCOMBE, C. S., and BINGHAM, W. F. "Men Who Have Accidents." *Personnel Journal* 6 (1927): 251–57.

YOST, C. P. "The Values of Total Fitness in Preventing Accidents." *National Safety Council Transactions* 23 (1961): 21.

4

traffic safety

The ability to transport persons and goods is a major factor in the security, comfort, and convenience of any modern nation. The motor vehicle provides a good part of this mobility. In many communities it is the only significant means of transportation. The motor vehicle also serves as the terminal operation for other transportation methods, such as by air, water, and rail, thereby contributing greatly to the efficiency of all transportation forms.

Many people fail to realize the extent to which our society is structured, economically and socially, around the motor vehicle industry. Consider these facts:

1. Nearly every job in the United States is dependent to some degree on the motor vehicle; some 13 million jobs—one in every six—are created by the motor vehicle industry.
2. Highway transportation of freight and people accounts for almost 17 percent of our gross national product.
3. More than 800,000 businesses hinge on motor vehicle use.
4. Motor vehicle users paid some $18 billion in special state and federal taxes in a recent year.
5. In the same year, the average state collected 19 percent of its tax revenue from motor vehicle users.[1]

[1] Motor Vehicle Manufacturers Association of the U.S., Inc., *Automobile Facts and Figures* (Detroit, 1972), pp. 55–59.

These facts make it easy to understand why the nation's economists are constantly concerned about fluctuations in the automotive market. A slowdown in the motor vehicle industry may cause layoffs for rubber workers in Akron, or a slowdown in steel mills in Pittsburgh and in the fabric industry in the Carolinas.[2] The economy of the United States, for good or bad, is tied directly to the motor vehicle.

The motor vehicle has restructured our lives in other ways. For example, it sparked the motel industry, with tremendous implications for hotels. It brought about drive-in restaurants, with important consequences for the food industry. The theater industry was reorganized with the advent of drive-in theaters made feasible by the automobile. Also, the nation's finance industry, a vital link in our economy, derives a huge portion of its income from the motor vehicle. Today's modern shopping centers exist largely because of the mobility provided by automobiles. Yet, vital as it is, the motor vehicle is only a single element in our highway transportation complex.

COMPONENTS OF OUR HIGHWAY TRANSPORTATION SYSTEM

Three distinct but highly interrelated components form our highway transportation system. They are:

1. The highway environment.
2. The vehicles that transport people and goods.
3. The people who function in the system.[3]

The efficiency, safety, and ultimate success of the system depend upon the proper functioning of each of the components. Its failure to operate correctly is the result of improper use, mismanagement, or poor highway design.[4] The consequences of these malfunctions are serious, since accidents often result from a breakdown in one or more of the system's components. In 1972, for example, highway transportation malfunctions caused approximately 56,600 deaths and more than 2,100,000 disabling injuries, or over 48 percent of the total accidental deaths in the United States during the same year. Aside from the untold human misery and suffering, the economic cost of these catastrophes was over 19 billion dollars.

[2] Motor Vehicle Manufacturers Assn., *Automobile Facts and Figures*, p. 61.
[3] *Driver Education for Illinois Youth*, The Office of the Superintendent of Public Instruction, Springfield, Illinois, 1972, p. 59.
[4] *Driver Education for Illinois Youth*, p. 51.

The current energy crisis necessitating lower speed limits and reduced travel should cause dramatic reductions in our highway death toll.
Further reductions may come about through mass transportation. Federal
highway statutes specify that urban areas with a population of 50,000 or
more must have a comprehensive transportation planning process in
operation to qualify for federal road funds. Without question, efficient
mass transportation systems would move more people faster and safer.

In the United States, the highway transportation complex comprises
about 4,000,000 miles of roads, streets, and highways of varying designs.
Operating within the system are more than 121,000,000 motor vehicles
of different shapes and sizes, traveling an estimated 1.25 trillion miles
annually.[5] An estimated 118,000,000 drivers,[6] all with different mental,
emotional, and physical characteristics, operate these vehicles. When you
add more than 71,000,000 pedacycles [7] and millions of pedestrians, neither
of which mix well in traffic patterns with motorized vehicles, it is easy to
understand why there is so much conflict in the system. Conflict means
time delays, as well as increased opportunity for accidents. Obviously
the problem deserves the attention and cooperation of every person in
this country.

To reduce highway accidents significantly, improvements must be
made in the system's components.[8] The "systems" concept requires a
multi-factoral approach involving many disciplines. The skills of highway
and automotive design engineers, human behavioral scientists, and people in the education field must all be combined. Experts from other areas,
such as medicine, biophysics, or human factors engineering, can also play
an important role.

Traffic engineering contributions such as limited access roads, elimination of grade crossings, road straightening, and better street lighting
have brought about many improvements.[9] These changes allow motor
vehicle operators to function more efficiently.

The automotive engineer, another vital contributor, must consider
both the driver and the road environment when designing an automobile.
Whenever possible, the human element with all its limitations must be
taken into account during the early stages of automobile design.[10]

The people who use the highway system represent the most chal-
lenging component for the reduction of accidents. There is general agreement that approximately 80 percent of accidents are caused by human

---

[5] National Safety Council, *Accident Facts 1973 Edition* (Chicago, 1973), p. 54.
[6] National Safety Council, *Accident Facts 1973*, p. 54.
[7] National Safety Council, *Accident Facts 1973*, p. 47.
[8] George Peters, "The Human Factors in Automobile Accidents," *International
Record of Medicine*, September 1958, p. 560.
[9] Peters, "The Human Factors," p. 560.
[10] Peters, "The Human Factors," p. 560.

error. In line with the systems approach we should consider methods of improving human behavior as it relates to the roadway and the vehicle. This requires making an analysis of the driving task. In this way, hopefully, we can determine how to develop and improve behavior while operating a motor vehicle. (See Chapter 9 for a sample task analysis of driving.)

ANALYSIS OF MOTOR VEHICLE CRASHES AND DEATHS

Motor vehicle death rates are generally expressed in three ways:

1. Deaths per 1,000,000 miles traveled.
2. Deaths per 100,000 population.
3. Deaths per 10,000 cars registered.

Figure 4-1 shows that between 1912 and 1972 motor vehicle deaths per 10,000 registered vehicles were reduced by 85 percent, from 33 to 5. Mileage figures were not available in 1912, but in 1972 there were about 30 times as many deaths as in 1910 and about 260 times as many vehicles on the highways, traveling faster and farther.

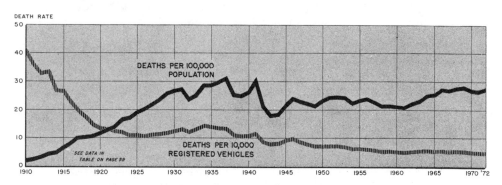

Figure 4-1. Trends in motor vehicle death rates. Reproduced from Accident Facts 1973 Edition, p. 41, courtesy of the National Safety Council.

Motor vehicle accidents claim many lives in all age groups. As Figure 4-2 illustrates, the death rate is highest among 15–24-year-olds. In fact, motor vehicle fatalities are the leading cause of death in this age group. According to National Safety Council data, approximately 80 percent of the victims are males.

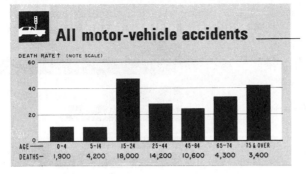

†Deaths per 100,000 population in each age group.

Figure 4-2. 1972 motor vehicle deaths by age groups. Reproduced from Accident Facts 1973 Edition, p. 42, courtesy of the National Safety Council.

Analysis of accident occurrence in relation to location yields some interesting figures. As is shown by the National Safety Council data in Table 4-1, motor vehicle accidents in rural places account for more than two-thirds of all motor vehicle fatalities, but nonfatal injuries occur more frequently in urban accidents. The proportions vary widely, however, for specific types of accidents: whereas, for example, only about one-third of all pedestrian fatalities occur in rural areas, more than 80 percent of deaths from noncollision accidents happen in such areas.

Another factor to be considered in accident analysis is the effect of nighttime driving on motor vehicle fatality frequency. Figure 4-3 makes it clear that although the number of deaths is only slightly higher at

Table 4-1. Motor vehicle deaths and injuries by type of accident, 1972.

Type of Accident	Deaths			Nonfatal Injuries		
	Total	Urban	Rural	Total	Urban	Rural
Total..........................	56,600	18,200	38,400	2,100,000	1,300,000	800,000
Collision with—						
Pedestrian......................	10,700	6,800	3,900	120,000*	105,000*	15,000*
Other motor vehicle............	24,200	5,900	18,300	1,570,000	1,020,000	550,000
Railroad train.................	1,500	400	1,100	5,000	2,000	3,000
Pedalcycle.....................	1,100	600	500	40,000	32,000	8,000
Animal, animal-drawn vehicle....	100	†	100	5,000	1,000	4,000
Fixed object...................	4,600	1,900	2,700	130,000	70,000	60,000
Noncollision...................	14,400	2,600	11,800	230,000	70,000	160,000

Source: National Safety Council estimates, based on reports from city and state traffic authorities.

†Less than 5.   *Injury totals not comparable to prior years due to classification change.

Reproduced from Accident Facts 1973 Edition, p. 45, courtesy of the National Safety Council.

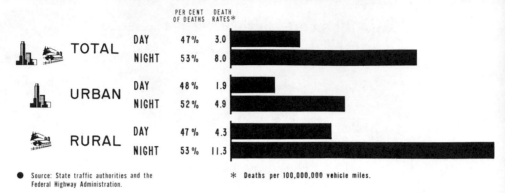

● Source: State traffic authorities and the
Federal Highway Administration.

* Deaths per 100,000,000 vehicle miles.

Figure 4-3. Deaths and death rates by day and night. Reproduced from Accident Facts 1973 Edition, p. 50, courtesy of the National Safety Council.

night, the *death rate*, computed as deaths per 100,000,000 vehicle miles, is considerably higher.[11] As the figure shows, this holds true for both urban and rural locations.

ETIOLOGY OF MOTOR VEHICLE CRASHES

Accidents are the result of various factors working in an interaction process. In an auto crash, sometimes the "entire cause" is mistakenly assigned to the "triggering" factor. A closer examination, however, usually reveals other factors that played an important role in the sequence of events leading to the accident itself.

An example might be some roadway object that causes a driver to attempt a sudden evasive maneuver with his vehicle in order to avoid the obstruction. In doing so, he loses control and crashes. The "entire cause" of the crash in this case is often assigned to the object or event that "triggered" the evasive maneuver. However, speed, alcohol, or other factors may have contributed just as much. In other words, the driver might have successfully completed the evasive procedure if he had not been traveling so fast or if he had had less to drink.

Deciding which elements are most responsible for an automobile crash is one of the most difficult problems in accident investigation. One must approach the etiology (assignment of cause) with caution.

We do know, however, that a few factors seem to have an unduly

[11] National Safety Council, *Accident Facts 1973*, p. 50.

high rate of involvement with motor vehicle crashes and their severity. These factors are:

1. Alcohol.
2. Human error or behavior.
3. Speed—too fast for conditions.
4. Vehicular defects.

There are various ways to classify the causes of automobile accidents. Alcohol and speed, for example, are actually not situational in nature, but are aggravating factors in many traffic situations. Using a wrong lane, which is included under human error, might actually be the result of the driver having too much alcohol. Following too close, also classified as human error, might not have resulted in an accident at lower speeds or in the absence of alcohol. There is no available data to assign accurate weights to speed and alcohol as they relate to various traffic situations. Both, however, greatly increase the risk inherent in all traffic situations.

alcohol

Special studies indicate that drinking is a contributing factor in at least one half of our fatal motor vehicle crashes.[12] Two of our society's characteristics make these crashes possible. We are a motor vehicle oriented society, and we are a drinking society. Therefore, it is inevitable that drinking and driving will occur simultaneously thousands of times each day.

There is no more conclusive evidence concerning accident cause-and-effect relationships than that involving alcohol and motor vehicle fatalities. Objective scientific evidence shows the effects on human behavior of various alcohol concentrations in the blood. But despite the scientific data available, there is still much confusion in this country about the effects of alcohol and alcoholism. Alcoholism is a disease characterized by loss of control over drinking. There are several dimensions to the alcohol problem, involving all of human experience—motivation, attitudes, values, and ecologic interactions within the environment.[13] Any safety worker will eventually have to deal with the problems of alcohol and alcoholism, since they are probably the nation's number one health hazard. All safety workers should further research the subject to

[12] National Safety Council, *Accident Facts 1973*, p. 52.
[13] C. R. Carroll, *Alcohol: Use, Non-Use, and Abuse* (Dubuque, Iowa: Wm. C. Brown Co., 1970), p. 1.

extend their understanding—thereby making themselves more capable safety workers as well as protecting their own health and well-being.

One of the most popular misconceptions concerning alcohol is that it is a stimulant. In fact, it is a depressant, and can be used as an anesthetic if a person so desires. The depressive effects of alcohol can be readily measured by techniques such as reaction time testing. However, many people do experience a very pleasant feeling after drinking a certain amount of alcohol. This fact undoubtedly accounts for the misconception that alcohol is a stimulant rather than a depressant.

Another misconception is that an alcoholic is a "skid-row bum," a derelict or society dropout who sleeps in alleyways and stays drunk every waking moment. That type of alcoholic represents only about from 3 to 5 percent of the total alcoholic population in this country. The confusion occurs because there are no standardized criteria to distinguish between alcoholics, problem drinkers, heavy drinkers, and social drinkers.

Alcoholism seems to be an insidious disease, at times asymptomatic. It apparently progresses through early, middle, and later stages. Sometimes this progression may take from 5 to 15 years or longer, during which time the person himself and others around him fail to recognize what is happening Most heavy drinkers and problem drinkers are potential alcoholics. Many alcoholics never reach the later stages, because they are killed accidentally or die prematurely from alcohol-related diseases.

It is difficult to estimate the incidence of alcoholism. Generally the primary statistics used are the number of drinkers who come to the attention of the police or who require medical attention for their problem. This means that most estimates are probably on the conservative side.[14] Some estimates place the number of alcoholics in the United States at approximately 9 million, with another 15 to 20 million classified as problem drinkers. In addition, there are millions of heavy drinkers and social drinkers. Approximately 93 million Americans drink to some extent.[15] These figures translate into millions of legally licensed drivers who, to greater or lesser degrees, have the potential to become involved in alcohol-related motor vehicle crashes.

As we know, there is scientific evidence of the effects of various blood levels of alcohol as they relate to traffic accidents and human behavior. The term "blood alcohol concentration" (BAC) refers to the amount of alcohol in the blood. This is expressed in terms of percentages: for example, a BAC of 0.05 percent would be 5 grams of alcohol per

[14] Kenneth L. Jones, Louis W. Shainberg, and Curtis O. Byer, *Drugs, Alcohol, and Tobacco* (San Francisco: Canfield Press, 1970), p. 71.

[15] Carroll, *Alcohol: Use, Non-Use, and Abuse*, p. 2.

100 milliliters of blood, and a reading of 0.10 percent would be equal to 10 grams of alcohol per 100 milliliters of blood. A reading of 0.50 would be 50 grams of alcohol per 100 milliliters of blood. A reading of 0.50 percent would occur in a 150-pound man if he drank approximately one fifth of 100-proof alcohol within one hour. A reading of 0.10 percent is enough for legal conviction for "driving under the influence" in many states. This would occur in a 150-pound man if he drank approximately five ounces of 100-proof liquor or five 8-ounce beers within one hour.

These estimates vary from person to person, depending on many factors such as rate of absorption and body weight. Oxidation rate is also very important, since alcohol accumulates in the body if ingested faster than it is oxidized. Thus, if a person ingests alcohol faster than one ounce per hour, over a period of time he will accumulate a very high BAC. Estimates of accumulation should be viewed with caution since the actual "effects" of accumulation also vary from person to person.

Research indicates that a BAC below 0.04 percent apparently does not threaten traffic safety. BACs over 0.04 percent, however, are definitely associated with increased accident involvement. In fact, the probability of becoming involved in an accident increases rapidly with BACs over 0.08 percent, and it is extremely high at concentrations over 0.15 percent.[16]

Figure 4-4 illustrates the probability of causing an accident in relation to the accumulated BAC. Although the data is based on rough estimates and should be used with extreme caution, the shape of the curve is consistent with accident involvement.

From this chart we can see that a person with a BAC of 0.15 percent is approximately 25 times more likely to have an accident than a person who has no alcohol in his bloodstream. At a BAC of 0.10 percent, a driver is approximately 7 times more likely to have an accident than a person with no alcohol involvement.

These are other interesting findings related to alcohol and driving:

1. High BACs are always associated with bad accident experience.
2. Drinking and driving are clearly associated with the frequent use or abuse of alcohol.
3. Many drivers with high BACs overestimate the number of drinks that it is safe to have before driving.[17]

Certain qualifications should be used when interpreting this type

[16] R. F. Borkenstein, R. F. Crowther, R. P. Shumate, W. B. Ziel, and R. Zylman, *The Role of the Drinking Driver in Traffic Accidents*, 4th ed. (Bloomington, Ind.: Department of Police Administration, Indiana University, 1969), p. 17.
[17] Borkenstein et al., *The Drinking Driver*, p. xviii.

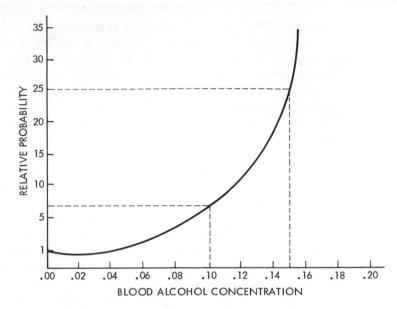

Figure 4-4. *The relative probability of causing an accident while drinking. Adapted from Borkenstein et al.,* The Role of the Drinking Driver in Traffic Accidents.

of data. The authors of the study suggest that if one is to use the data he should examine the limitations listed in the study iself.[18]

Other research tends to confirm the findings of the above study. However, W. L. Carlson, in a separate report, added more conclusions.

1. There is a higher concentration of high BAC drivers in the early morning hours. Drivers with BACs of 0.10 percent constitute only 2 to 3 percent of the driving population before midnight, but jump to 8 percent after midnight.
2. High BAC drivers tend to drive on less heavily traveled roads during the early morning hours.[19]

SUGGESTED ALCOHOL COUNTERMEASURES. Before we can effectively fight drinking while driving, we must overcome public apathy. Why does the public fail to respond to such overwhelming evidence? The answer, as with all other accidents, lies in the "isolation factor." For example, the total of 56,000 traffic fatalities in a single year represents one person

[18] Borkenstein et al., *The Drinking Driver*, p. xvii.
[19] W. L. Carlson, "Alcohol Usage of the Nighttime Driver," *Journal of Safety Research* 4, No. 1 (March 1972): 24.

killed for every 3,500 of the total population. If one half of the traffic fatalities are alcohol related, this represents one person in every 7,000 population. On the average, then, a city with a population of 7,000 will lose two people per year in traffic crashes, but only one will be alcohol related.

Also it would appear that a BAC of 0.10 percent as a basis for legal conviction of driving under the influence is a very liberal interpretation. It certainly is beyond a "reasonable doubt," which is the legal criterion for conviction.

Research indicates that less than 0.2 percent of the drivers on the road have BACs of 0.15 percent or higher.[20] Estimates from urban studies on alcohol and traffic crashes indicate that 90 percent of the alcohol-related fatal crashes could be eliminated by removing that 0.2 percent from the traffic flow.[21]

R. F. Borkenstein rightfully contends that this means a decision could be made to concentrate on removing BACs in excess of 0.15 percent, based on social science research. This would have the effect of substituting a well-defined goal for a shot-gun approach.[22] He estimates that one in every 500 drivers has a BAC of over 0.15 percent on an around-the-clock basis, with the heaviest concentration from 8 P.M. to 3 A.M. He also estimates that a city of 50,000 people will have 200,000 violations of drinking/driving laws per year.[23]

One of the greatest problems in this area is the 20–24-year-old age group. Drivers in this age bracket have an alarming arrest record for aggressive driving provoked by alcohol and are "over represented" in alcohol-related traffic crashes.[24] This is a very serious public health problem—the death rate in this age group would show a dramatic reduction if it were not for alcohol-related traffic crashes.

Since more drinking violations occur at night, it seems logical to concentrate law enforcement during the nighttime hours. Carlson recommends increased nighttime enforcement in areas of low traffic density.[25]

Stepped-up enforcement procedures would likely be effective against the social drinker. However, the problem drinker and the alcoholic represent a social problem that would probably need efforts other than increased enforcement. Increased education on the subject should be helpful, especially with younger drivers.

[20] R. F. Borkenstein, "A Panoramic View of Alcohol, Drugs, and Traffic Safety," *Police Magazine*, July 1972, p. 9.
[21] P. M. Hurst, "Estimating the Effectiveness of Blood Alcohol Limits," *Behavioral Research in Highway Safety* 1 (1970): 87–89.
[22] Borkenstein, "A Panoramic View," p. 9.
[23] Borkenstein, "A Panoramic View," p. 11.
[24] Borkenstein, "A Panoramic View," p. 12.
[25] Carlson, "Alcohol Usage," p. 18.

Perhaps we must find different methods of transportation to remove the high BAC from traffic. The alcohol–traffic crash problem needs immediate attention, at least with experimental countermeasures and adequate research. More comprehensive enforcement procdures coupled with more severe penalties are definitely indicated. We might impose punitive action for the first offense, and a much stronger penalty for the second offense. The number of arrests for alcohol-related traffic accidents should also be greatly increased.

human error and behavior

Improper driving behavior and human error are leading causes of motor vehicle accidents. They include using the wrong lane, following too closely, failing to yield the right of way, failing to stop at signals, making improper turns, and much more. As we know, speed and alcohol aggravate all these situations.

Table 4-2, based on National Safety Council data for 1972, lists the most common kinds of improper driving that contributed to accidents. Of course, most accidents involve road and vehicle conditions as well as driver behavior, but the correction of improper driving practices could help considerably in reducing the number of accidents.

Table 4-2. Improper driving reported in accidents, 1972.

Kind of Improper Driving	Fatal Accidents			Injury Accidents			All Accidents*		
	Total	Urban	Rural	Total	Urban	Rural	Total	Urban	Rural
Total......................	100.0%	100.0%	100.0%	100.0%	100.0%	100.0%	100.0%	100.0%	100.0%
Improper driving................	78.5	76.4	79.2	87.8	83.5	91.0	88.4	85.8	92.8
Speed too fast†................	26.9	20.1	28.4	19.3	11.5	25.1	14.6	8.2	24.9
Right of way..................	13.1	21.1	11.1	20.3	30.1	13.2	20.2	24.2	13.8
Failed to yield...............	9.1	14.7	7.7	14.5	21.0	9.8	14.9	17.7	10.3
Passed stop sign............	2.8	2.9	2.8	2.9	3.7	2.3	2.6	2.8	2.4
Disregarded signal..........	1.2	3.5	0.6	2.9	5.4	1.1	2.7	3.7	1.1
Drove left of center.........	12.4	5.8	14.2	4.3	2.4	5.8	3.6	2.3	5.8
Improper overtaking..........	1.9	2.0	1.9	1.9	1.4	2.3	3.0	3.1	2.7
Made improper turn...........	0.6	1.0	0.6	1.3	2.1	0.7	3.0	4.1	1.1
Followed too closely..........	1.0	2.5	0.6	8.4	9.9	7.3	11.6	14.3	7.1
Other improper driving........	22.6	23.9	22.4	32.3	26.1	36.6	32.4	29.6	37.4
No improper driving stated.......	21.5	23.6	20.8	12.2	16.5	9.0	11.6	14.2	7.2

Source: Reports of state and city traffic authorities, as follows: Urban-43 cities; Rural-13 states; Total—NSC estimates based on Urban and Rural reports.
*Principally property damage accidents, but also includes fatal and injury accidents.
†Includes "speed too fast for conditions."

Reproduced from Accident Facts 1973 Edition, p. 48, courtesy of the National Safety Council.

Human error is an elusive target in preventing accidents because it is dependent upon so many factors that are not readily discernable. The great variations in personality and behavior severely limit our ability to correct human error in accidents.

speed

The speed capability of the modern automobile is a perfect example of how automotive engineering has outpaced road design. It is also an example of how automotive engineering goes beyond human capabilities for safe driving.

Speed itself is a relative factor. Within reasonable limits, you can be safe even at relatively high speeds. However, speed becomes dangerous when the vehicle is being driven *too fast for conditions*. The amount of traffic, weather and road conditions, and the physical and mental condition of the driver are all important considerations in deciding how fast to drive.

However, once an accident or crash does occur, speed is a critical factor in determining just how severe it will be. The severity of accidents goes up dramatically with higher speed, because force of impact increases so rapidly with increases in speed.

Most people tend to drive at speeds that are both safe and legal. As we know, factors such as alcohol or mental attitude influence driving speed. It is also influenced by the posted speed limit. Yet, the posted speed limit is a commonly misunderstood element in selecting driving speed. The legal posted speed limit *does not* necessarily indicate a safe speed at that particular time. Conditions at the time *always* determine what is and what is not a safe speed.

Driving too slow can also be dangerous, when other traffic is moving faster or in instances where traffic is very light and cars are free to move at higher speeds. In either case a slow-moving vehicle does not mix well with the regular flow of traffic. It is extremely difficult for one driver to judge how fast he is approaching another vehicle moving in the same direction.

Today most posted speed limits are set at the 85th percentile—the speed at which 85 percent of the cars are traveling safely with minimum accident frequency. Most modern automobiles are designed to operate more efficiently and safely at moderate speeds.

motor vehicle defects

Isolated studies indicate that automobile defects may be an important cause of accidents. (Comprehensive national statistics on motor vehicle defects in traffic accidents are not available.) Reports from Kansas and Washington, for example, indicate that bad tires comprised 74 percent of the defects in vehicles involved in fatal accidents, and 47 percent of the defects in all accidents. Brakes were defective in 9 percent of the fatal accidents, and in 25 percent of all accidents.[26]

The ultimate blame for continuing to drive a vehicle with known defects such as bad tires or faulty brakes must be charged to the operator, either as poor knowledges or faulty attitudes. The operator of a motor vehicle should know whether the tires or brakes are safe or not. In a brake failure, the driver is usually given ample warning in the form of a grabbing brake, a low braking pedal, a soft braking pedal, or other signs. A careful visual inspection of the tires will usually show if they are bad or not. To operate a motor vehicle with known defects of any kind is both senseless and dangerous.

Without comprehensive data, it is difficult to decide the worth of state automobile inspection laws. However, if automobile defects are known causes of accidents, it stands to reason that inspection laws, if properly enforced, could reduce the accident rate. The standardization of all laws, including motor vehicle inspection, is long past due.

THE ACTION PROGRAM FOR HIGHWAY SAFETY

The Action Program for Highway Safety, sometimes called the "President's Action Program," is an official guide for states to use in developing their own highway safety programs. Established at the President's Highway Safety Conference in 1946,[27] it was to set the guidelines for the nation's traffic safety for years to come.

Although the program was revised in 1949 and 1960, the basic principles remain the same.[28] The original eight guidelines have been expanded to include eleven areas: [29]

1. Laws and Ordinances.
2. Traffic Accident Records.
3. Education.
4. Engineering.
5. Motor Vehicle Administration.
6. Police Traffic Supervision.
7. Traffic Courts.
8. Public Information.
9. Research.

[26] National Safety Council, *Accident Facts 1973*, p. 57.
[27] The President's Committee for Traffic Safety, *Highway Safety Action Program* (Washington, D. C., 1966), p. 4.
[28] The President's Committee, *Highway Safety Action Program*, p. 5.
[29] The President's Committee, *Highway Safety Action Program*, p. 10.

10. Health, Medical Care, and Transportation of the Injured.
11. Organized Citizen Support.

FEDERAL LEGISLATION

In 1966 federal intervention into highway safety was strengthened through two legislative acts—The National Traffic and Motor Vehicle Act and The Highway Safety Act. The first empowered the federal government to establish standards for design and construction of safe vehicles.[30] In effect, this centralized, at the federal level, control over the original design of motor vehicles. States could no longer set individual standards. The second act empowered the federal government to assist state and local governments in their safety programs.[31]

From such legislation, the Department of Transportation (DOT) was created in 1966. An agency of the department is the National Highway Traffic Safety Administration (NHTSA), which has established standards in the following areas of highway safety:

1. Periodic Motor Vehicle Inspection.
2. Motor Vehicle Registration.
3. Motorcycle Safety.
4. Driver Education.
5. Driver Licensing.
6. Codes and Laws.
7. Alcohol in Relation to Highway Safety.
8. Traffic Courts.
9. Identification and Surveillance of Accident Locations.
10. Traffic Records.
11. Emergency Medical Services.
12. Highway Design, Construction, and Maintenance.
13. Traffic Control Devices.
14. Pedestrian Safety.
15. Police Traffic Services.
16. Debris Hazard Control and Cleanup.[32]

These areas are indicative of the scope and importance of the highway traffic safety problem in this country. Obviously there are no

[30] The President's Task Force on Highway Safety, *Mobility without Mayhem* (Washington, D. C.: U. S. Government Printing Office, 1970), p. 1.
[31] The President's Task Force, *Mobility without Mayhem*, p. 1.
[32] National Highway Safety Bureau, *Highway Safety Program Standards* (Washington, D. C., n.d.).

easy solutions. The traffic safety problem challenges the ability of the most competent men and women in the nation.

THE THREE E's OF TRAFFIC SAFETY

The traffic safety problem is categorized into three distinct areas:

1. Enforcement.
2. Engineering.
3. Education.

traffic law enforcement

The purpose of traffic law enforcement is to protect the public. It helps to control those few violators who would do harm to the majority through misuse of motor vehicles. Enforcement gives meaning to traffic signs and other regulatory mechanisms. It has a proven direct effect on driver behavior. Good traffic law enforcement reduces traffic accidents and saves lives.

Effective traffic law enforcement is dependent upon quality work in several areas. A breakdown in any one of them may cause deterioration of the entire enforcement process. The areas having the most effect on enforcement are:

1. Legislation.
2. Motor Vehicle Administration.
3. Police Departments.
4. Traffic Courts.

LEGISLATION. Legislation provides the legal foundation and offers guidelines for the entire enforcement procedure. The growth of the traffic problem makes it important that laws and ordinances be based on sound, realistic principles and be clearly stated. They should be uniform throughout all states and communities.[33]

National concern for effective legislation and enforcement is not new. Herbert Hoover called the first National Conference on Street and Highway Safety in 1924. The result was the Uniform Motor Vehicle Code and the Model Traffic Ordinance,[34] both regarded as the best in

[33] The President's Committee, *Highway Safety Action Program*, p. 10.
[34] C. T. Adams, *Law Enforcement*, 2nd ed. (Englewood Cliffs, N. J.: Prentice-Hall, Inc., © 1973), p. 201.

regulatory standards. Yet, we still do not have uniform traffic laws across the nation. Motorists and pedestrians alike often become confused when they travel from state to state.

The use of the motor vehicle has increased dramatically in recent years. Automotive and road engineering have made significant gains. But legislation has failed to keep pace. Existing laws need a complete review to determine which are obsolete and what new laws are needed to make each state uniform. A prime concern should be the development of uniform speed limits for different classes of highways.

MOTOR VEHICLE ADMINISTRATION. Motor vehicle administration includes driver licensing, driver improvement, vehicle inspection, titling, registration, and financial responsibility. Because so much detailed information is needed in these areas, motor vehicle administration is by nature a cumbersome process. Although computers have greatly streamlined the work, a wide disparity still exists in the administrative methods used across the country.

The licensing of drivers and motor vehicles alone makes administration extremely important. Yet, due to lack of identification, the enforcement of suspended or revoked driver licenses is virtually non-existent.[35] Methods must be developed to provide this identification if we are to make our highways safer. Good driver improvement schools must be developed on a state-by-state basis, with appropriate referral procedures set up in cooperation with the courts.

POLICE DEPARTMENTS. Police responsibility in traffic enforcement and management covers three areas:

1. Traffic direction and control.
2. Accident investigation.
3. Law enforcement.[36]

Modern police departments work more efficiently through the use of electronic computers and radar surveillance equipment. One effective technique is selective enforcement—using enforcement on the types of violations that are causing accidents, at times when and places where the accidents are actually occurring. To be effective, this technique uses much statistical data for proper scheduling and deployment.[37] And it is effective, for accident rates go down as enforcement in high accident areas is increased.

[35] The President's Task Force, *Mobility without Mayhem*, p. 39.
[36] The President's Committee, *Highway Safety Action Program*, p. 32.
[37] J. W. Rutherford, "Reducing Traffic Accidents Through Selective Enforcement," *The Police Chief*, May 1971, p. 8.

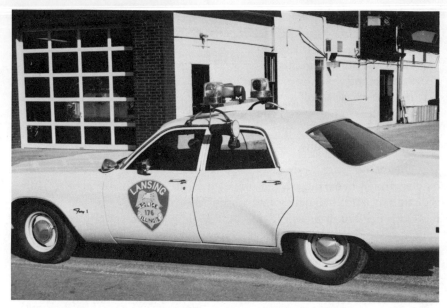

Figure 4-5. *A police radar speed-detection device mounted on a police vehicle. Photo courtesy of the Lansing, Illinois, Police Department.*

The level, quality, and uniformity of traffic enforcement must be raised. The courts should allow the police to use devices that can automatically record vehicle violations. The use of presently available electronic and photographic technology should help to resolve questions of fact.[38] Massive public education campaigns are needed to develop better public support and understanding of our police departments. Improved recruitment and selection techniques are needed for police personnel. More thorough training procedures must be set up, with ample opportunity for participation in refresher courses.

The accident forms presently used by police departments might also be revised to make them compatible with the needs of traffic engineers who are working to correct hazardous locations. Standardizing these forms nationally could prove invaluable for research purposes. Theoretically they might provide now unknown clues, such as the possible effects of humidity, temperature, and other variables as they relate to traffic accidents.

TRAFFIC COURTS. Many of our traffic courts are so overloaded that they have literally turned into cafeteria-style operations. These courts should be classified into specialized areas for uniformity, and there should

[38] The President's Task Force, *Mobility without Mayhem*, p. 39.

also be more uniformity in the assessment of penalties. Effective ways must be found to stop the "fix" in the courts, so that penalties will be applied equally to all. In fact, the entire area of enforcement needs to be researched thoroughly and streamlined to become a more useful tool in saving lives and reducing accidents. The following is a relevant quotation from Howard Pyle prior to his retirement as president of the National Safety Council:

> Not only is it important to design and enact the best laws possible but we must also develop a knowledgeable, sophisticated, and concerned police and judicial law enforcement system. By the coordination of their efforts and the sharing of their resources, the laws we seek today may become the life savers of tomorrow.[39]

traffic engineering

Traffic engineering concerns the planning, geometric design, and traffic operations of roads, streets, highways, and abutting lands. Its purpose is to promote the safe, efficient, and convenient movement of persons and goods.[40]

As a profession, traffic engineering can be traced to the beginnings of automobile production in the late nineteenth century. However, there are examples of specific traffic engineering practices dating back to the early days of the Roman Empire, which dates from 27 B.C. For instance, the Romans enforced one-way traffic for chariots and would not allow them in certain business sections during specified hours. They also had off-street chariot parking. There is evidence that pavement markings were used on a road leading from Mexico City around 1600 A.D. In the United States the first center line appeared on a street in Wayne County, Michigan, in 1911. The first traffic signal was put up in Houston, Texas, in 1921, followed a year later by the first coordinated signal system.[41]

The traffic engineering profession itself is still young and is characterized by a shortage of highly trained specialists. Many large cities still do not have such a highly trained individual on their staff, and as a result are being denied a critical traffic safety service.

The traffic engineer must consider problems of a physical nature and human behavior problems of both driver and pedestrian, with all of the resulting interrelationships. This means that the traffic engineer must

---

[39] Howard Pyle, "Traffic Safety Is Low Man on the Totem Pole," *Traffic Safety Magazine*, January 1972, p. 36.

[40] L. J. Pignataro, *Traffic Engineering—Theory and Practice* (Englewood Cliffs, N. J.: Prentice-Hall, Inc., © 1973), p. 2.

[41] Pignataro, *Traffic Engineering—Theory and Practice*, p. 2.

have a knowledge of highway design as it relates to the basic characteristics of the vehicles on our streets and highways, and to the individuals
operating those vehicles.

Carefully obtained facts are the basis for all decisions and planning.
For traffic engineers to obtain the necessary facts for their decisions, they
must become dependent upon studies from several areas, including:

1. Road users.
2. Vehicles.
3. Speed, travel time, and delay.
4. Traffic volume counts.
5. Origin and destination.
6. Capacity.
7. Parking.
8. Accidents.
9. Public transit.[42]

Without question, traffic engineering is making a significant impact
on the reduction of accidents on the nation's highways. Our present
interstate system is a case in point for illustrating the effect of good
highway design on highway safety.

About 31,900 miles of the Interstate System were completed to full
or acceptable standards by the end of 1972. They carried an estimated
195,370,000,000 miles of travel. If deaths with this amount of travel had
occurred at a rate of 4.5, the rate on all of the nation's highways in 1972,
compared with a preliminary estimate of about 2.5 for the portion of
the completed interstate, there would have been approximately 3,900
more deaths during the year than actually occurred.[43]

It is estimated that a primary highway of modern design will have
an accident rate 30 to 40 percent lower than that of a primary highway
designed 30 to 40 years ago.[44] This is further evidence of the effectiveness
of our advancing technology of highway design.

Some examples of good traffic engineering that are readily noticeable
(some can be seen in Figure 4-6) are such things as:

1. Correction of hazardous locations.
2. Channelization of traffic.
3. Rush-hour controls.
4. One-way streets.

[42] Pignataro, *Traffic Engineering—Theory and Practice*, p. 4.
[43] National Safety Council, *Accident Facts 1973*, p. 44.
[44] The President's Task Force, *Mobility without Mayhem*, p. 27.

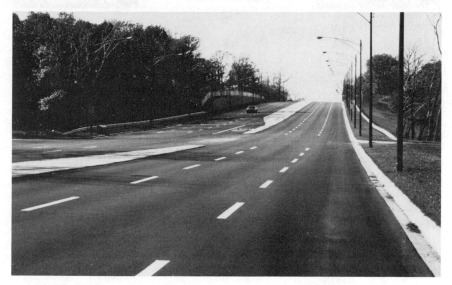

Figure 4-6. *An example of good traffic engineering. Note the channelization, street lighting, and offset left-turn lane. Photo courtesy of the Bureau of Streets and Sanitation, Chicago, Illinois.*

5. Traffic-signal systems.
6. Pavement markings.
7. Street lighting.

Research indicates that highway lighting cuts down on nighttime accidents. Cities should study their peak traffic hours closely and determine time schedules that allow more daylight hours during peak traffic hours. With our present technology, we could develop highway lighting systems automatically controlled by light detection devices that would trigger their operation according to the lighting needs at any given time.

Figure 4-7 illustrates the new road signs that are being used today —another example of improved engineering techniques.

education

The goal of driver and traffic safety education is to develop citizens who will be safe and responsible users of our highway transportation system. The concept should be comprehensive and should include all of the users of the highway transportation system, pedestrians and pedacyclists as well as the motor vehicle operators.

Private and community orientated programs deal with traffic safety education, in addition to the massive educational programs conducted in

TWO WAY TRAFFIC — W

DIVIDED HIGHWAY — W

DIVIDED HIGHWAY ENDS — W

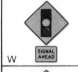

LOW CLEARANCE — W

MERGE — W

SIGNAL AHEAD — W

SLIPPERY WHEN WET — W

HILL — W

KEEP RIGHT — R

NO PASSING ZONE — W

RED
Regulatory

YELLOW
Warning

BLUE
Services

GREEN
Guidance

ORANGE
Construction

BROWN
Recreation & Scenic

●

INTERSTATE NUMBERING SYSTEM

ONE- AND TWO-DIGIT SIGNS:
(through routes)

Even numbered signs are East-West routes
Odd numbered signs are North-South routes

THREE-DIGIT SIGNS:

First digit even: loop through or around a city
First digit odd: spur route.

TWO WAY TRAFFIC — W

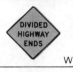

DIVIDED HIGHWAY — W

DIVIDED HIGHWAY ENDS — W

LOW CLEARANCE 12 FT 6 IN — W

MERGING TRAFFIC — W

SIGNAL AHEAD — W

SLIPPERY WHEN WET — W

HILL — W

KEEP RIGHT — R

DO NOT PASS — R

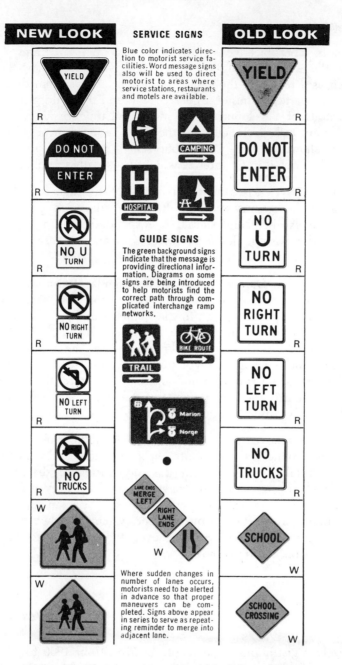

NEW LOOK

SERVICE SIGNS

Blue color indicates direction to motorist service facilities. Word message signs also will be used to direct motorist to areas where service stations, restaurants and motels are available.

OLD LOOK

GUIDE SIGNS

The green background signs indicate that the message is providing directional information. Diagrams on some signs are being introduced to help motorists find the correct path through complicated interchange ramp networks.

Where sudden changes in number of lanes occurs, motorists need to be alerted in advance so that proper maneuvers can be completed. Signs above appear in series to serve as repeating reminder to merge into adjacent lane.

Figure 4-7. The new versus the old look in road signs.

our schools. The objectives of all driver education programs should be based on the essential requirements of safe driving. Analyzing the driving task itself as it relates to the highway transportation system should reveal the desired characteristics of a good driver, and it should provide insight into methods of developing these specific characteristics. (An analysis of the driving task, included with the driver education programs in our schools, is shown on page 175. Public school driver education programs are treated in detail in Chapter 9, which deals with school safety.)

ADULT DRIVER EDUCATION PROGRAMS. Many high schools and colleges across the country offer adult driver education programs. They have proven excellent and should be expanded, offering opportunities for those who wish to learn to drive, as well as those who wish to improve their driving skills.

COMMERCIAL DRIVING SCHOOLS. Thousands of commercial schools are in operation across the country, some good and some poor. One common weakness seems to be in the quantity and quality of the classroom instruction programs. Another weakness is the inadequate training of their behind-the-wheel instructors. However, many states are now maintaining more stringent regulations for these schools. If they train high school students and are reimbursed by the state, they should meet the same standards and requirements of the state's high schools in terms of teacher qualification and quality of curriculum.

DRIVER IMPROVEMENT SCHOOLS. Chronic traffic violators need help in changing driving behavior. State bar associations and police organizations should take the lead, with the cooperation of driver education groups, in setting up driver improvement schools. They would be very helpful to our court system for referral purposes. Such an approach would add meaning and prestige to our present system of driver improvement schools. If persistent traffic violators cannot be reeducated, they should be removed from the traffic flow.

MOTORCYCLE SAFETY

Motorcycle registrations increased from 575,497 in 1960 to 3,787,000 in 1972,[45] a six-fold rise. This rapid growth in such a short time has made the motorcycle an important factor in our highway transportation system.

The mileage death rate (per 100,000,000 miles of motorcycle travel)

[45] National Safety Council, *Accident Facts 1973*, p. 56.

is 17, compared with an overall motor vehicle death rate of 4.5. The overall motor vehicle death rate includes pedestrians and non-occupants, as well as occupant deaths.[46] The high death rate from motorcycle accidents indicates an immediate need for increased emphasis on enforcement and on motorcycle safety education.

Motorcycles are an economical means of transportation, a fact often especially important to young people. And fifty percent of all motorcycle crashes involve youthful operators with less than two years of experience.[47]

The characteristics of motorcycles make them more liable to accidents—they do not have the built-in stability of other motor vehicles. Stability must be provided by the operator. Motorcycles are more hazardous in a crash than other motor vehicles—the operator of a motorcycle as well as any passengers riding with him have more exposure than people occupying other types of vehicles.[48] Motorcycles are light in comparison to automobiles, and are capable of developing very high speeds. All of these characteristics make it necessary for an operator of a motorcycle to maintain a high level of performance.

Unless we develop educational programs in motorcycle safety, it is inevitable that the number of deaths and the death rates from motorcycles will continue to increase. Regardless of how one personally feels about motorcycles and their use, we must institute programs aimed at reducing accidents involving motorcycles.

One area that makes such accident reduction difficult involves licensing and testing for licenses. This must be taken into account by all motor vehicle administrators, and proper practices must be established for licensing and testing of the operators.

Some people feel that the most likely place for motorcycle education is in driver education programs at the high school and college levels. This would mean that high schools and colleges would have to reevaluate their programs and staffs. Additional specialized training would be needed for instructors.

In 1968 the National Commission on Safety Education of the National Education Association initiated steps that resulted in guidelines and policies for motorcycle education. Many states are adopting these into their high school driver education programs. Since we can expect increased numbers of motorcycles to appear in our highway system, present highway safety program standards must be implemented as a minimal program in all states.

---

[46] National Safety Council, *Accident Facts 1973*, p. 56.
[47] National Education Association, *Policies and Guidelines for Motorcycle Education* (Washington, D. C., n.d.), p. 1.
[48] National Education Association, *Motorcycle Education*, p. 2.

PEDACYCLE SAFETY

Since 1935 the number of pedacycle–motor vehicle deaths has more than doubled. The number of pedacycles in use has increased twentyfold; therefore the death rate (per 100,000 pedacycles) has decreased to approximately one-tenth the 1935 rate. Persons 15 years and older accounted for one half the deaths in 1972 compared to about one fifth in 1960. This reflects the increase in usage by older age groups. There were 71.4 million pedacycles in use in 1972.[49]

The increase in the number of deaths from pedacycles and their increasing use indicate a need for more pedacycle programs in our communities. There are several organizations with suitable programs and materials available. Many pedacyclists are presently in schools, so our efforts in pedacycle safety should be increased especially at the lower grade levels. Communitywide programs should be expanded to reach the older cyclists.

According to a National Safety Council survey, collisions between motor vehicles and bicycles occur about as follows:

1. 50 percent occur at intersections.
2. 70 percent happen during the daylight hours.
3. 80 percent of the bicyclists are violating traffic laws at the time of the accident.
4. 50 percent of the motor vehicle–bicycle accidents involve a violation on the part of the motor vehicle operator.
5. 20 percent of the bicycles involved in accidents have some mechanical defect.[50]

The most common traffic violations by cyclists are:

1. Riding in the middle of the street.
2. Failure to yield right of way. (In some cases the cyclist does not see the car. In some cases he intentionally infringes on the motorist's right of way.)
3. Riding too fast for conditions.
4. Disregard of traffic signs or signals.
5. Riding against the flow of traffic.
6. Improper turning.[51]

---

[49] National Safety Council, *Accident Facts 1973*, p. 47.
[50] National Safety Council, *Bicycles*, Safety Education Data Sheet No. 1 rev. (Chicago, n.d.), p. 1.
[51] National Safety Council, *Bicycles*, p. 1.

Other injuries are caused by falls on slippery surfaces, deep ruts, sand, or gravel; collision with pedestrians or fixed objects; falls from defective or overloaded bikes.[52] Figure 4-8 illustrates some of the safety and maintenance factors of bicycles.

rules for safe bicycling

1. Observe all traffic regulations. Always be ready to yield the right of way: you will never win in a contest with a car.
2. Keep to the right, as close to the curb as practicable. Ride in a straight line, single file.
3. If you must drive at night, have a white headlight in good working order and a red reflector on the rear. Wear white or light-colored clothing.
4. Have and use a horn or bell for signalling. No sirens!
5. Always give pedestrians the right of way. Know local regulations regarding driving on sidewalks. If you must use the sidewalk, it is best to walk your bike in congested areas.
6. Watch for parked cars pulling out into traffic, and for car doors that open suddenly.
7. Never hitch onto other vehicles, stunt or race in traffic.
8. Never carry riders. Packages should be carried in a basket or rack. Except when signalling, hands should be on handlebars at all times.
9. Be sure your bike is in safe mechanical condition.
10. Slow down at all intersections. Look both ways: left, right, then left again before crossing.
11. Use proper hand signals when turning, stopping, or slowing. Always be aware of traffic behind as well as in front of you.
12. Mature bike drivers do not "horse around." Bike driving is fun —accidents are not! [53]

PEDESTRIAN SAFETY

Pedestrian traffic is an element in sharp conflict with vehicular traffic. The consequence is a high accident rate and delayed traffic.[54]

Pedestrian accidents resulted in 10,700 deaths in 1972. This represents almost 19 percent of the total motor vehicle related fatalities. Over one-half of these deaths are in the 0–14, and the 65 year and-older,

---

[52] National Safety Council, *Bicycles*, p. 2.
[53] National Safety Council, *Bicycles*, p. 7.
[54] Pignataro, *Traffic Engineering—Theory and Practice*, p. 252.

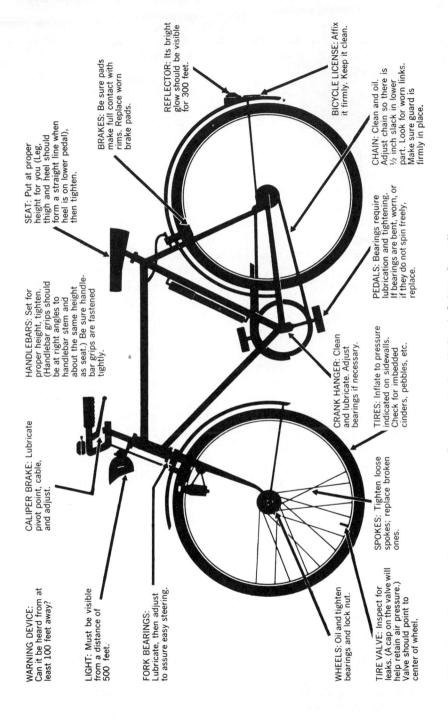

Figure 4-8. Bicycle maintenance factors. Courtesy of the National Safety Council.

REFLECTOR: Its bright glow should be visible for 300 feet.

BICYCLE LICENSE: Affix it firmly. Keep it clean.

BRAKES: Be sure pads make full contact with rims. Replace worn brake pads.

SEAT: Put at proper height for you (Leg, thigh and heel should form a straight line when heel is on lower pedal), then tighten.

CHAIN: Clean and oil. Adjust chain so there is ½ inch slack in lower part. Look for worn links. Make sure guard is firmly in place.

HANDLEBARS: Set for proper height, tighten. (Handlebar grips should be at right angles to handlebar stem and about the same height as seat.) Be sure handlebar grips are fastened tightly.

PEDALS: Bearings require lubrication and tightening. If bearings are bent, worn, or if they do not spin freely, replace.

CRANK HANGER: Clean and lubricate. Adjust bearings if necessary.

CALIPER BRAKE: Lubricate pivot point, cable, and adjust.

TIRES: Inflate to pressure indicated on sidewalls. Check for imbedded cinders, pebbles, etc.

WARNING DEVICE: Can it be heard from at least 100 feet away?

SPOKES: Tighten loose spokes; replace broken ones.

LIGHT: Must be visible from a distance of 500 feet.

WHEELS: Oil and tighten bearings and lock nut.

FORK BEARINGS: Lubricate, then adjust to assure easy steering.

TIRE VALVE: Inspect for leaks. (A cap on the valve will help retain air pressure.) Valve should point to center of wheel.

74

groups.[55] This indicates that a large percentage of pedestrian accidents involve non-drivers, people who undoubtedly do not have an awareness of the problems of maneuvering and stopping a car.

Typically, peak pedestrian and motor vehicle traffic coincide. This is usually during morning, noon, and evening rush hours.[56] Seven out of ten pedestrian deaths occur when people cross or enter streets.[57] Intersections are especially hazardous. Among the older age groups, fatalities seem to be predominately males who frequently have been drinking.

Four factors apparently combine to add to the seriousness of the pedestrian safety problem:

1. Speed differentials between pedestrians and motor vehicles do not allow them to mix well in traffic patterns.
2. The peak hours of vehicular movement and pedestrian movement coincide.
3. Alcohol is a factor with the motor vehicle operator and with the older age groups of pedestrians.
4. Many pedestrians are non-drivers and thus do not appreciate the problems involved in the operation of a motor vehicle.[58]

The high frequency of pedestrian accidents points to the need for increased safety education efforts at all levels. (See Chapter 9, "School Safety.") Presently recommended standards on pedestrian safety should be implemented as the minimum essential practice in all states. At heavy traffic intersections, pedestrian and vehicular traffic could be separated by elevated or depressed pedestrian walkways.[59]

SUMMARY

The motor vehicle has revolutionized many aspects of modern society. It has given us a necessary and vital mobility. With these advantages, however, have come over 2,000,000 fatalities and many more millions of disabling injuries.

The motor vehicle accident problem is complex because it involves the thinking and behavior of millions of people. It also involves the interaction of these people with vehicles of various shapes and sizes operating on roadways of different designs.

[55] National Safety Council, *Accident Facts 1973*, p. 42.
[56] Pignataro, *Traffic Engineering—Theory and Practice*, pp. 256–57.
[57] National Safety Council, *Accident Facts 1973*, p. 55.
[58] The President's Task Force, *Mobility without Mayhem*, p. 43.
[59] Pignataro, *Traffic Engineering—Theory and Practice*, p. 257.

We are now seeing a coordinated effort on a national scale to reduce this terrible accident rate. The use of new "systems" techniques will provide a more balanced and multifactoral approach. The problem requires the cooperation of every member of our society.

Research indicates that strong countermeasures, especially concerning alcohol-related crashes, are sorely needed. This could provide one of the quickest inroads into solving the problem. Increased driver education programs will also help.

The motor vehicle problem will surely become larger and more complex. We can expect increases in both the number of drivers and vehicles in the immediate future. Effective mass transportation planning offers great promise of diminishing the traffic safety problem in both rural and urban areas.

SUGGESTED STUDENT ACTIVITIES

1. Write a paper defending or attacking motorcycle education as a part of driver education in high schools and colleges.

2. Prepare a 20-minute speech on the "systems" concept as related to our highway transportation system.

3. Design a model of the driving task.

4. Make a complete traffic movement analysis at a busy intersection. Count the number of right turns, left turns, straight ahead movements, and pedestrian movements.

5. Plan a program for pedestrian education in your community.

6. Prepare a paper on effective countermeasures for alcohol-related motor vehicle crashes.

7. Prepare a research paper on ways we might improve or streamline our traffic courts.

8. Hold a panel discussion in your class with students representing the areas of engineering, enforcement, and education.

9. Plan and execute a 10-minute teaching demonstration concerning some phase of driver education. Develop your own teaching aids.

10. Visit your police department. Prepare a map showing the high accident locations in your community.

BIBLIOGRAPHY

ADAMS, C. T. *Law Enforcement.* 2nd ed. Englewood Cliffs, N. J.: Prentice-Hall, Inc., 1968.

BORKENSTEIN, R. F. "A Panoramic View of Alcohol, Drugs, and Traffic Safety." *Police Magazine,* July 1972, pp. 9–12.

BORKENSTEIN, R. F.; CROWTHER, R. F.; SHUMATE, R. P.; ZIEL, W. B.; and ZYLMAN, R. *The Role of the Drinking Driver in Traffic Accidents.* 4th ed. Bloomington, Ind.: Department of Police Administration, Indiana University, 1969.

CARLSON, W. L. "Alcohol Usage of the Nighttime Driver." *Journal of Safety Research* 4, No. 1 (March 1972): 24.

CARROLL, C. R. *Alcohol: Use, Non-Use and Abuse.* Dubuque, Iowa: Wm. C. Brown Co., 1970.

HURST, P. M. "Estimating the Effectiveness of Blood Alcohol Limits." *Behavioral Research in Highway Safety* 1 (1970): 87-99.

JONES, KENNETH L.; SHAINBERG, LOUIS W.; and BYER, CURTIS O. *Drugs, Alcohol, and Tobacco.* San Francisco: Canfield Press, 1970.

MOTOR VEHICLE MANUFACTURERS ASSOCIATION OF THE U. S., INC. *Automobile Facts and Figures.* Detroit, 1972.

NATIONAL EDUCATION ASSOCIATION. *Policies and Guidelines for Motorcycle Education.* Washington, D. C., n.d.

NATIONAL HIGHWAY SAFETY BUREAU. *Highway Safety Program Standards.* Washington, D. C., n.d.

NATIONAL SAFETY COUNCIL. *Accident Facts 1973 Edition.* Chicago, 1973.

————. *Bicycles.* Safety Education Data Sheet No. 1 rev. Chicago, n.d.

OFFICE OF THE SUPERINTENDENT OF PUBLIC INSTRUCTION. *Driver Education for Illinois Youth.* Springfield, Illinois, 1972.

PETERS, GEORGE. "The Human Factors in Automobile Accidents." *International Record of Medicine,* September 1968, p. 560.

PIGNATARO, L. J. *Traffic Engineering—Theory and Practice.* Englewood Cliffs, N. J.: Prentice-Hall, Inc., 1973.

THE PRESIDENT'S COMMITTEE FOR TRAFFIC SAFETY. *Highway Safety Action Program.* Washington, D. C.

THE PRESIDENT'S TASK FORCE ON HIGHWAY SAFETY. *Mobility without Mayhem.* Washington, D. C.: U. S. Government Printing Office, 1970.

PYLE, HOWARD. "Traffic Safety Is Low Man on the Totem Pole." *Traffic Safety Magazine,* January 1972, p. ·36.

RUTHERFORD, J. W. "Reducing Traffic Accidents Through Selective Enforcement." *The Police Chief,* May 1971, p. 8.

5

home safety

Most people think of the home as a refuge from the hazards of the highway, the office or factory, and other areas of high risk. Accident statistics, however, do not support that view. The home is actually one of the more dangerous places you can be.

In 1972, for example, there were 27,000 accidental deaths in the home and approximately 4,200,000 disabling injuries.[1] This means that about 23 percent of the total accidental deaths in this country occurred in the home or on the home premises, and during the same period 1 in every 50 persons in the United States suffered a disabling injury in or around the home.

A more meaningful analysis of home accident statistics might be to consider a city of 7,000 people. At present rates that city will average almost two deaths per year in home accidents, and disabling injuries will strike another 140 people.

The cost of home accidents is presently running at least 3 billion dollars per year! And this figure includes only lost wages, medical expenses, and insurance administrative costs. It does not include property-damage losses, for which fires alone total 800 million dollars per year.[2]

[1] National Safety Council, *Accident Facts 1973 Edition* (Chicago, 1973), p. 79.
[2] National Safety Council, *Accident Facts 1973*, p. 79.

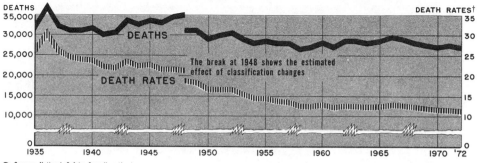

Figure 5-1. Trends in home accidental deaths and death rates. Reproduced from Accident Facts 1973 Edition, p. 79, courtesy of the National Safety Council.

Figure 5-1 illustrates the downward trend in home death rates in recent years. Some comfort might be found in the fact that the 1972 death rate of 11.3 per 100,000 population was 52 percent below the rate for 1935. Actually, however, there were more deaths from home accidents in 1972 than there were in 1935 (after adjusting for the 1948 change in method of classification). There were also more people, especially in the age groups most susceptible to fatal accidents—children under five years of age and persons over 65. Although the decrease in accidental death rates may seem encouraging, the high accident rates in the home represent a serious safety problem in our society.

The alarming statistics on home accidents become more so when reviewing the home environment. Today's modern home contains many conveniences and much equipment that create high accident potential. It also contains an array of chemicals in the form of polishes, detergents, pesticides, fertilizers, and others. In recent years modern medicine has added a variety of medicines that are dangerous when misused. Alcohol and drug use have aggravated the situation.

Living in this sophisticated environment are people who are not well trained in the use of these conveniences. They are therefore highly susceptible to human error and misjudgment through carelessness and poor habits, skills, and attitudes. This combination of factors creates a series of high-risk situations.

A modern kitchen may be convenient, but note in Figure 5-2 how human error has created a potential accident through the incorrect placement of cooking utensils. A bad burn or scald can easily result.

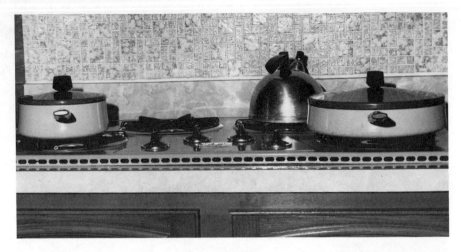

Figure 5-2. Utensils improperly placed on a stove. Photo courtesy of Jack Green, Sr.

UPGRADING HOME SAFETY PROGRAMS

If home accident rates are to be reduced, we must improve both the quality and quantity of home safety programs. Until now these programs have been largely in the form of home inspections for fire or other hazards. If found, the hazards are removed, but there is little or no emphasis on education and training to reduce human error and unsafe acts. Thus home safety programs in a sense are at the level of industrial programs of 50 years ago, when the emphasis was on hazard removal, not human error. In addition, there has been little or no follow-up on these programs, and no evaluation to provide a basis for long-range planning. As in most poor safety programs, the lack of accident data is apparent.

The many different types of home accidents present special problems in their prevention. For example, industry can focus attention on a given department and on specific accident situations. It can then remove the hazards and initiate effective training and education programs with follow-up and evaluation procedures. The many kinds of home accidents in scattered locations make this specialized treatment impossible.

To be successful, home accident prevention programs should:

1. Have a starting point, with some community agency—a service club, a safety council, or any interested group—assuming the responsibility.

2. Have close coordination of all groups that become involved.
3. Perform surveys of home accidents.
4. Develop a communitywide accident record system of home accidents for analysis and planning purposes. This will require the cooperation of doctors, clinics, and hospitals.
5. Initiate planned programs on a long-range basis.
6. Perform regular home inspection programs with follow-up procedures. (A home safety checklist is included at the end of this chapter.)
7. Provide more constant use of education campaigns through the schools and on a home-to-home basis.
8. Develop more effective use of the mass media.
9. Perform yearly evaluations over a period of years to determine the effectiveness of the efforts and to realign priorities.

Obviously such an approach requires extensive organization and effort. Many civic clubs are searching for projects, needing only to be prodded into action. If home safety programs do not begin in some way and become effective, we can reasonably expect government action, indicated by the federal government's interest in other safety areas. The Product Safety Commission is a definite step toward government intervention into home safety.

FALLS IN AND AROUND THE HOME

Falls have always been a major cause of accidental death in homes and elsewhere. They are outranked only by automobile accidents as a cause of accidental death.[3] In a recent year 9,800 people lost their lives through falls in or around the home. That figure includes falls from one level to another, such as falling on stairs, from ladders, or from the roof. It also includes falls on the same level, such as falling on the floor, ground, or sidewalk.[4]

As we know, the death rate from falls goes up significantly with older age groups. Of the above 9,800 deaths, 1,000 were in the age group 45–64; 1,400 were in the 65–74-year-old group; and 6,700 in the age group 75 and older.[5]

There are many proximate and contributing factors involved in falls. Like other accidents they are the result of unsafe conditions or unsafe

[3] National Safety Council, *Falls*, Safety Education Data Sheet No. 5 (Chicago, n.d.).
[4] National Safety Council, *Accident Facts 1973*, p. 80.
[5] National Safety Council, *Accident Facts 1973*, p. 80.

acts, or a combination of the two.[6] Unsafe conditions include such things as slippery floors or surfaces, loose wires or cords, and toys, pets, or even children. Unsafe acts are a bigger cause. They involve things that people either do or fail to do—walking with their hands in their pockets on slippery surfaces (and thereby being unable to protect themselves if they do fall); failing to check a ladder for faulty rungs or proper placement; and failing to remove snow, ice, or mud from trafficked surfaces. These human errors may be caused by illness, poor vision, inexperience, fatigue, dizziness, emotional distress, lack of skill, poor judgment and foresight, and intoxication.[7]

Figure 5-3 shows an anatomy of a fall in the home, listing many but not all of the elements that may be involved in such an accident. It divides the causes into "unsafe conditions" and "unsafe acts," adding the all-important timing factor.

Most falls in and around the home could be prevented if people would take the necessary precautions, including an analysis of the home environment followed by proper planning to remove or compensate for the hazards. (This simple task is especially necessary in homes which include elderly people.) Figure 5-4 shows the steps that should be taken to reduce the possibilities of falls in the home.

FIRES IN THE HOME

Fires in the home, as well as burns and deaths resulting from them, are responsible for the loss of almost 6,000 lives each year in the United States. These deaths are mainly caused by carelessness, which allows a fire to get started, and by poor pre-fire planning, which hinders escape and promotes the rapid spread of the fire.

The age groups most susceptible to death from home fires are the 0–4 group and those 45 and older. The very young, the very old, the handicapped, and the ill present special problems in home fires because of their relative immobility under emergency conditions.

Fire records clearly indicate that the first eight weeks of living in a home, old or new, are the highest ignition-hazard period.[8] The new tenant is unfamiliar with the surroundings and oftentimes overloads circuits, misuses fireplaces, or the like.

Figure 5-5 shows suggested steps in fire prevention programming

[6] National Safety Council, *Falls*, Data Sheet No. 5.

[7] National Safety Council, "Falls," *Farm Safety Review*, July–August 1973, p. 8.

[8] Rexford Wilson, "A Fire Safe House," *Farm Safety Review*, November–December 1972, p. 3.

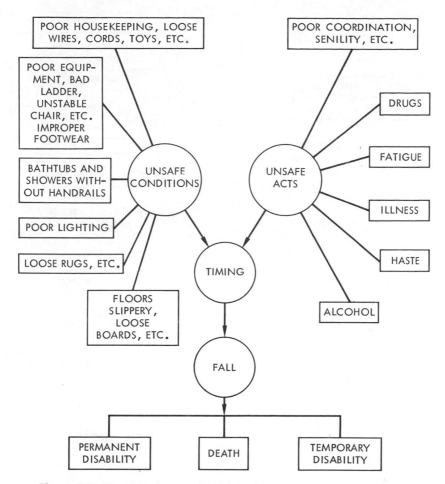

Figure 5-3. *The anatomy of a fall in the home.*

for the home. The first step is to check the home to determine existing fire hazards. People should take advantage of fire department inspections, and initiate their own surveys as well.

Once the survey has been completed, the process of eliminating hazards should begin immediately. Good housekeeping includes removing such things as rubbish and old newspapers, especially on stairways, near furnaces, and in closets, and keeping matches out of reach of young children. No one should smoke in bed, and all rooms should be equipped with fire-resistant ashtrays. Dry leaves and rubbish are yard hazards and should be removed. Garages should be checked for improper storage of paints, pesticides, and other flammable liquids. Poor wiring, overloaded

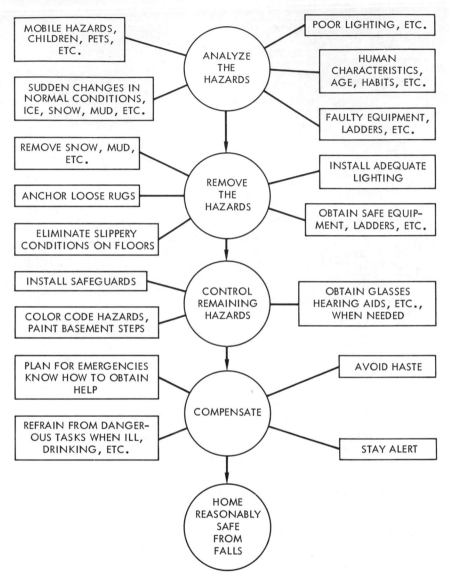

Figure 5-4. *Countermeasures against falls in the home.*

circuits, and inadequate or poorly made extension cords are electrical hazards.

Cooking involves numerous hazards. Provisions should be made for controlling grease fires, and drapes or other flammable material near a stove should be removed.

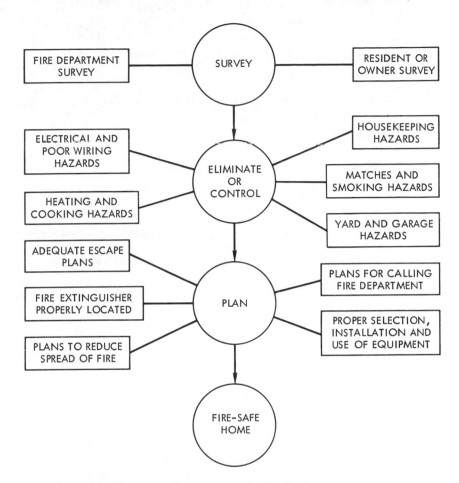

Figure 5-5. Fire prevention programming in the home.

Heating hazards occur when a furnace is not kept in good operating condition, and when flues are not well cleaned or repaired. Heating equipment should be checked annually by qualified people.

Equipment and appliances in the home should be properly selected, installed, and used. Good planning also calls for fire extinguishers located near exits. Adequate escape plans are vitally important. In the event of fire two things are immediately necessary, in this order—get everyone out of the house, and call the fire department.

Plans for an escape from a home fire should include the following:

1. Draw up a home floor plan and decide on escape routes.
2. Select alternate escape routes from every room in the house. Use

windows if necessary; you cannot count on using a stairway or hall.

3. Instruct the family in the use of windows leading to another roof, such as a porch. You may have to wait there until the fire department arrives.
4. Have ladders handy. Fire escape ladders are available and can be stored in accessible places.
5. Designate a meeting place so that all members can be accounted for. This is extremely important.
6. Hold fire drills and practice your plan.[9]

Some additional fire safety tips include sleeping with bedroom doors closed. If you suspect fire, check the door for evidence of heat. If in doubt, open the door slightly by placing one hand at the top and one on the knob, and brace your foot against the bottom. If there is a fire, super-heated air can create enough pressure to knock you down when you open the door.

Every family member should know how to call the fire department and how to turn in an alarm (*before* trying to extinguish the fire alone). Be sure everyone knows the location of the alarm nearest your home. The importance of calling the fire department as soon as everyone is out of the house cannot be overemphasized. The quicker you receive professional help, the less chance for the fire to get completely out of control. When calling the fire department:

1. Remain calm; think before you call.
2. Report the number of your house.
3. Report the street or road on which the house is located.
4. Report any unusual markings or things that might identify your house.
5. Report the number from which the call is being made.

See Chapter 13 for a more extensive discussion of fire safety, the chemistry of fires, and the types of extinguishers suitable for different fires.

SUFFOCATION

Suffocation accidents are responsible for over 3,000 deaths each year, with about 1,250 of them in the 0–4 age group. These accidents are classi-

[9] National Safety Council, *Planned Fire Escape For Your Family,* pamphlet (Chicago, n.d.).

fied in two ways—suffocation by ingestion and mechanical suffocation. Suffocation by ingestion includes death from accidentally ingesting or inhaling an object or food that obstructs the respiratory passages. Mechanical suffocation includes death from smothering by bed clothes, thin plastic materials, or the like, as well as death from cave-ins or confinement in closed spaces, and strangulation.[10]

One of the more common and more deadly objects that people—especially children—inhale is the dried bean. Once it is in the air passages, the bean absorbs moisture and increases greatly in size. Children using bean shooters are often subject to this when they inhale deeply while preparing to discharge the bean from the tube. The deep inhalation sucks the bean into the air passages. Peanuts are another dangerous object when inhaled, and should be removed immediately by a physician. Children especially may swallow almost any small object. (See Figure 5-6.)

When an object lodges in the throat, the throat muscles go into convulsions. This is nature's way of expelling a foreign object. Usually the resulting coughing and gagging will expel the object. If not, other measures must be taken immediately—any good first-aid book will list them. Read and memorize them; they may save a life.

Parents should be extremely careful of allowing small children to play with any kind of plastic bag, especially if it is large enough to fit over the child's head. Caution should also be used when choosing crib bedding. If parents took proper precautions, most of the mechanical suffocation deaths of small children could be prevented.

POISONING BY SOLIDS AND LIQUIDS

Poisoning by solids and liquids is responsible for slightly over 3,000 deaths per year, including deaths from drugs, medicines, shellfish, and mushrooms, as well as from the commonly recognized poisons. This figure does not include poisonings from spoiled foods, salmonella and others, which are classified as disease deaths.[11]

The chemical substances and mixtures in the home, including medications, cleaning agents, polishing agents, and exterminating agents,[12] must be properly stored, preferably under lock when not in use, to keep them away from children. They can be deadly poisonous.

Common causes of childhood poisonings are aspirin, pain relievers,

[10] National Safety Council, *Accident Facts 1973*, p. 80.
[11] National Safety Council, *Accident Facts 1973*, p. 81.
[12] National Safety Council, *Solid and Liquid Poisons*, Safety Education Data Sheet No. 21 rev. (Chicago, n.d.).

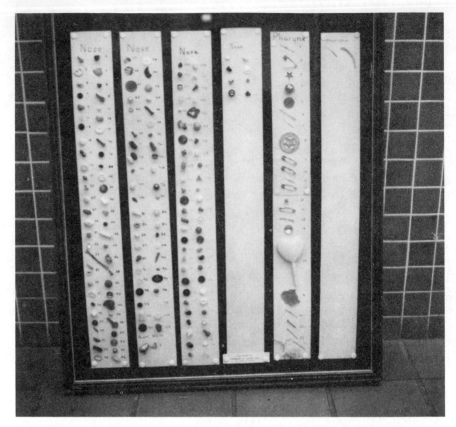

Figure 5-6. Actual objects removed from people's noses, throats, etc. Photo courtesy of Arthur J. Kuhn, M.D., Hammond Clinic, Munster, Indiana.

laxatives, and sedatives—all generally found in the medicine chest.[13] It might be well to purchase a medicine cabinet that can be opened easily by adults but with difficulty by children. There are several types available.

Accidental-poisoning victims require immediate first aid. A general rule to remember is "hurry and dilute." In some cases it is desirable to induce vomiting; however, this is not necessarily so in all poisoning cases. A mistake in treatment could be fatal. Read a first-aid manual on poisons. One simple precaution that would speed up first aid for a poisoning victim would be to post the information shown in Figure 5-7 on the inside of the medicine cabinet and near a phone.

Poison control centers are located in various cities throughout the

[13] National Safety Council, *Solid and Liquid Poisons.*

EMERGENCY TELEPHONE NUMBERS

Physician's Office _____ Home _____

Poison Control Center _____

Hospital _____

Pharmacist _____

Rescue Squad _____

Fire Department _____

Police Department _____

Figure 5-7. *Information useful in an emergency.*

United States. Check with your physician to see if inquiries should be made by the physician or if they can be made directly to the poison control center.

The physician or the poison control center will want to know what chemicals are in the poison that was swallowed, before advising first-aid procedures. This makes it imperative to keep the label and have it handy when reporting the emergency. To give adequate treatment, the physician must get accurate information and get it rapidly.

POISONING BY GASES AND VAPORS

Poisoning by gases and vapors accounts for approximately 1,100 deaths per year. Most such deaths involve carbon monoxide, resulting from faulty cooking stoves or heating equipment and idling motor vehicles. Gas poisonings that result from fires are classified as fire deaths.[14]

Allowing a car to idle inside a garage is an extremely bad policy. There is immediate danger both in the garage itself and in the car if it is driven shortly thereafter. Although not classified as a home death, one common cause of carbon monoxide poisoning occurs when people load the trunk of a car and are unable to close the lid completely. Traveling on a highway, a car with an open trunk lid apparently creates a vacuum, and the carbon monoxide fumes are sucked directly into the car from the rear. Never drive a car with an open trunk without adequate ventilation inside the car.

[14] National Safety Council, *Solid and Liquid Poisons.*

FIREARMS

Firearms account for approximately 2,300 accidental deaths each year. Approximately 60 percent (1,400) of them occur in the home or on the premises.[15] Most of these deaths could be avoided by taking a few simple precautions.

People purchase guns for many different reasons, from personal protection to hunting and recreational shooting. Many people keep loaded firearms in their bedrooms for protection against possible intruders. All too often a person shoots a member of his own family in the dark. It is highly questionable whether one should keep a gun in the bedroom for such purposes since it probably would provoke the intruder into shooting.

Most accidental firearm deaths are the result of improper storage, careless handling, or poor cleaning. A surprising number of deaths result from people handling guns that they thought were not loaded. Under no circumstances should people handle guns and ammunition without adequate training.

Even a toy rifle can be dangerous. A 10-year-old Chicago boy, after discovering ammunition in his home, loaded a bullet into his toy gun and pulled the trigger. Both the bullet and the gun exploded, sending several pieces of steel into his hand.[16]

To make your home free from the possibility of firearm accidents, follow these rules:

1. Never keep a loaded gun in the house or anywhere on the premises.
2. Keep all guns out of the reach of children and preferably locked up. If the guns are kept in a display rack, the rack should be locked and the key carefully hidden away.
3. All ammunition should be stored separately from the gun, and also locked up.
4. Never allow a gun to be brought into the house without checking both the magazine and the chamber yourself to be sure it is not loaded.

Two other points to remember: never point a gun—loaded or unloaded—at anyone or anything unless you intend to use it; and always

15 National Safety Council, *Accident Facts 1973*, p. 81.
16 National Safety Council, "Trigger to Tragedy," *Family Safety Magazine,* Winter 1969, p. 23.

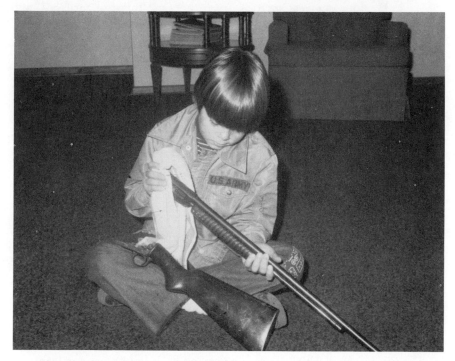

Figure 5-8. A small boy cleaning a gun. This boy has been properly trained in the techniques of cleaning a gun. Note the dismantled gun. Photo courtesy of Joseph C. Krutzsch.

break a gun muzzle before handing the gun to someone else. This simple courtesy may save a life.

DANGEROUS EQUIPMENT IN THE HOME

Hundreds of thousands of injuries every year are associated with equipment that is commonly used in the home. An estimate from the Injury Control Program of the U.S. Public Health Services lists 12 household equipment items that are most often involved in home accidents. The victims are usually children, frequently "helpful" or curious boys of five and under. The accidents usually result from misusing the equipment.

The 12 types of equipment thought responsible for most injuries from home accidents are:

1. Home machinery, such as electric drills, sanders, planers, and various power saws.

2. Heating devices, such as space heaters, full-size furnaces, and floor furnace grates.
3. Clothes wringers.
4. Power mowers (thrown objects).
5. Cooking stoves.
6. Skillets (burns from hot handles and poured or splattering grease).
7. Incinerators (especially dangerous because of burns associated with starting fluids).
8. Glass doors (children running through glass doors they thought were open).
9. Appliance cords (children pull cords and are struck by the appliance or its contents).
10. Sockets and extensions (children chew on cords and stick bobby pins into sockets).
11. Sun lamps (overtime exposure to skin and failure to use eye protection).
12. Pilots and burners (explosions from paint and solvent vapors near the flames).[17]

other home accidents

Approximately 2,500 deaths are caused each year by home accidents other than those already mentioned. They include accidental deaths from such things as drowning, electric currents, explosive materials, and blows from falling objects. The 0–4 and the 75 and older age groups are involved in one half of these fatal accidents.

HOME SAFETY CHECKLIST [18]

kitchen

Do you—   Yes   No

1. Use nonskid wax on your floors?   _____   _____

2. Have stove and sink areas well lighted?   _____   _____

3. Turn pot handles away from stove front, but not over another burner?   _____   _____

[17] National Safety Council, "The Dangerous Dozen," *Family Safety Magazine,* Fall 1967, p. 17.
[18] Reprinted courtesy of the National Safety Council.

4. Wipe up spills immediately?   ____ ____

5. Open oven door before turning on gas to light it manually?   ____ ____

6. Follow directions when using your pressure cooker?   ____ ____

7. Have a rack or compartmented tray for sharp knives?   ____ ____

8. Keep electric appliances away from sink area and make sure your hands are dry before operating them?   ____ ____

9. Have at least two hot-dish holders near the stove?   ____ ____

10. Have metal containers for waste paper and cans?   ____ ____

11. Use a step stool when reaching into high cupboards?   ____ ____

12. Clean range exhaust hood and duct frequently?   ____ ____

13. Have emergency phone numbers handy to your telephone (police, fire, doctor, utilities)?   ____ ____

living, dining, bedroom

Do you—   Yes   No

1. Have nonskid backing on small rugs, and avoid use at top of stairs?   ____ ____

2. Keep traffic areas and exits clear of furniture and obstructions?   ____ ____

3. Use a screen in front of your fireplace?   ____ ____

4. Have plenty of wall outlets for lamps and appliances; avoid octopus connections?   ____ ____

5. Have lamp within reach of bed?   ____ ____

garage and driveway

Do you—   Yes   No

1. Have your garage in order: tools in place, floor clean, flammable liquids stored in safety cans?   ____ ____

2. Have your garage well lighted with switches at doors?   ____ ____

3. Set "Park" or hand brake and lock car when you leave it outside?

4. Check area around car before backing?   ____ ____

workshop

Do you—   Yes   No

1. Keep paint thinners and solvents in metal containers?   _____   _____
2. Keep power tools disconnected or switches locked when not in use?   _____   _____
3. Store oily rags in air-tight metal cans?   _____   _____
4. Keep tools out of the reach of small children?   _____   _____
5. Have workshop well ventilated and work areas well lighted?   _____   _____
6. Have a dry powder, carbon dioxide or all-purpose fire extinguisher handy?   _____   _____
7. Ground power tools before using them?   _____   _____
8. Use safety glasses?   _____   _____
9. Keep power tool guards in place?   _____   _____

bathroom

Do you—   Yes   No

1. Have nonskid mats or textured surfaces in tubs and showers?   _____   _____
2. Have a sturdy grab bar for your tub or shower?   _____   _____
3. Have medicines clearly labeled, and read the labels before taking any medicine?   _____   _____
4. Keep medicines stored safely out of the reach of small children?   _____   _____
5. Dry your hands before using electrical appliances— and never operate them when you're in the bathtub?   _____   _____
6. Avoid using hair sprays near open flame or when smoking?   _____   _____

stairways

Do you—   Yes   No

1. Have sturdy handrails for outside steps and inside closed stairways?   _____   _____

2. Have attic stairs well lighted?

3. Have sturdy bannisters on open stairs and stairwells?

4. Keep childrens' toys off stairs?

5. Avoid using stairways for storage areas?

6. Have stairs well lighted with switches at top and bottom?

7. Keep treads, nosing, and carpeting in good repair?

storage area

Do you—   Yes   No

1. Avoid using your basement, attic or utility room for a "dumping ground," especially for combustible materials?

2. Have attic floored if used for storage?

3. Keep rubbish and wastepaper in metal containers?

basement or utility room

Do you—   Yes   No

1. Know where your main gas and water valves are located and how to close them?

2. Have gas and water lines distinctly tagged so they can be quickly identified?

3. Know how to light the pilot light on your furnace and water heater?

4. Have your gas dryer vented to the outside (if designed for outside venting)?

5. Call the gas company if you suspect a leaky valve or pipe?

6. Know where your main electrical switch is and how to turn it off?

7. Have extra fuses on hand and pull the main switch before changing a fuse?

8. Determine what has caused a fuse to blow and eliminate the cause before replacing the fuse?

9. Know the maximum load each of your electrical circuits can safely carry and avoid overloading them?   ____ ____

10. Have fuses or circuit breakers labeled to identify outlets and fixtures they protect?   ____ ____

11. Keep combustibles away from hot light bulbs?   ____ ____

12. Have a 20-ampere line to safely carry the heavy load needed to operate kitchen appliances such as electric grills, waffle irons, rotisseries?

13. Have washer and dryer electrically grounded?   ____ ____

14. Have a metal ironing board or an asbestos pad for a wooden one?   ____ ____

15. Keep cleaning fluids, drain openers, ammonia, and similar items locked up or out of the reach of small children?   ____ ____

outside

Do you—   Yes   No

1. Return garden tools to their storage racks after use?   ____ ____

2. Get help for heavy or difficult jobs?   ____ ____

3. Limit the time you work in the hot sun (severe sunburn or sunstroke is serious business)?   ____ ____

4. Keep children and pets at a safe distance while operating your power mower?   ____ ____

5. Shut off the mower when cleaning, adjusting or emptying grass catcher, and never refuel when motor is hot?   ____ ____

6. Use charcoal lighter fluid to light your outdoor grill (never gasoline)?   ____ ____

7. Keep ladders in good shape—replace loose rungs, worn ladder shoes, frayed ropes on extension ladders?   ____ ____

8. Use extra care putting up screens or storm windows when you're on a ladder, especially in windy weather?   ____ ____

9. Keep your trash burner covered when using it?   ____ ____

10. Repair broken walks and driveways?   ____ ____

11. Have clotheslines high enough to clear pedestrian traffic?   ____ ____

12. Have your television antenna grounded?   ____ ____

SUMMARY

Accident records definitely mark the home environment as a dangerous place. Since most individuals spend most of their time in this environment, exposure rates may be high.

Today's standard of living, made possible by increased technology and increased medical knowledge, has allowed a variety of gadgets and medicines to permeate a society that is generally unprepared to utilize these advances in a safe manner.

Many unsafe acts combine with a high number of unsafe conditions to produce high-risk situations in the home. Carelessness, lack of knowledge or training, faulty attitudes, and poor skills aggravate the home accident situation.

There is a definite need for well-planned, well-coordinated communitywide home safety programs using all forms of safety. Home safety programs should be given high priority, with the emphasis on falls. Programs to date have been scattered and for the most part poorly organized with little utilization of the mass media. Follow-up and accurate evaluation are a must for any community efforts focusing on home safety.

SUGGESTED STUDENT ACTIVITIES

1. Survey your own home for hazards. Follow this with a program designed to reduce or control these hazards.
2. Draw up a home fire escape plan for use in emergencies.
3. Practice your home fire escape plan.
4. Hold a family training meeting to be sure all members of the family who are old enough to understand know how to shut off water, gas, and electricity.
5. Draw plans for a potential communitywide home safety program.
6. Make a task analysis of mowing the yard.
7. Analyze a home accident that has occurred in your home, or that of a friend, and determine the unsafe acts and unsafe conditions that combined to cause the accident.
8. Inspect your home medicine cabinet and discard old and unused medicines and other potential hazards.
9. Visit a poison control center and see the types of calls they get. Report back to your class.
10. Invite a member of the fire department to speak before your class on home fire safety.

BIBLIOGRAPHY

NATIONAL SAFETY COUNCIL. *Accident Facts 1973 Edition.* Chicago, 1973.

————. "The Dangerous Dozen." *Family Safety Magazine,* Fall 1967.

————. "Falls." *Farm Safety Review,* July–August 1973.

————. *Falls.* Safety Education Data Sheet No. 5. Chicago, n.d.

————. "The Hazard Hunter." Pamphlet. Chicago, 1968.

————. *Planned Fire Escape for Your Family.* Pamphlet. Chicago, n.d.

————. *Solid and Liquid Poisons.* Safety Education Data Sheet No. 21 rev. Chicago, n.d.

————. "Trigger to Tragedy." *Family Safety Magazine,* Winter 1969.

WILSON, REXFORD. "A Fire Safe House." *Farm Safety Review,* November–December 1972.

6

occupational safety

EARLY WORKING CONDITIONS IN THE UNITED STATES

The industrial safety movement did not develop simultaneously with the industrial revolution; instead, it began many years later. Working conditions in the early part of the 19th century were characterized by poor sanitation facilities, poor lighting, poor ventilation, and poor equipment with inadequate safeguards. The fatigue factor, caused by excessively long working hours, also contributed to high accident rates in industry. How high they really were is not known, but undoubtedly they were appalling judged by today's standards. At the time there was no organized collection of accident data, and so there was no particular means of bringing the problem to the attention of the public.[1]

It was not until after 1850 that some legislation was passed concerning industrial safety. Even at this point, workmen's compensation laws were still more than 60 years away; injury cases were handled by "common law" in the courts. This meant that the employee had little, if any, chance to be compensated for an industrial injury.

Employers had four good defenses available to them under the "common law" system:

[1] R. H. Simonds and J. V. Grimaldi, *Safety Management* (Homewood, Ill.: Richard D. Irwin, Inc., 1963), p. 17.

1. The employer was not negligent.
2. Another employee was responsible or contributed to the cause of the accident.
3. The employee through his own negligence contributed to the accident.
4. The employee was aware of the hazards involved and still accepted employment.[2]

Employers also had the benefit of the best legal minds of the day. If an employee did sue, he would likely end up with no compensation for his injury and lose the cost of the lawsuit in the process. Also, he was putting his job in jeopardy.

The earliest legislation took the form of authority to investigate and regulate, but laws of this type were unpopular and proved hard to enforce. In 1867 Massachusetts, one of the leading states in the area of safety legislation, enacted a law requiring the appointment of factory inspectors. A few years later it passed the first enforceable law for a 10-hour per day working maximum. In 1877 it enacted legislation requiring the guarding of dangerous machinery.[3]

Laws which attempted to place some liability upon the employer were slow in evolving. Some humanitarian employers might offer jobs as night watchmen or janitors to people who had lost an arm or an eye, but there was no legal requirement that they do so. It was not until 1885 that Alabama passed the first state legislation defining employer liability. Massachusetts followed in 1887.[4] Although these laws defining employer liability did not have much effect at the time, they probably laid the groundwork for the future development of workmen's compensation laws. At least the principle was being developed that the employer should share in the cost of the accidents and should compensate for the injury to the extent of his liability.

Apparently the steel industry was in the forefront of future safety efforts, as evidenced by a statement in 1906 by Judge Elbert Gary, president of United States Steel Corporation:

> The United States Steel Corporation expects its subsidiary companies to make every effort practicable to prevent injury to its employees. Expenditures necessary for such purposes will be authorized. Nothing which will add to the protection of the workers should be neglected.[5]

[2] Dan Petersen, *Techniques of Safety Management* (New York: McGraw-Hill Book Co., 1971), p. 10.
[3] H. W. Heinrich, *Industrial Accident Prevention* (New York: McGraw-Hill Book Co., 1959), p. 425.
[4] Heinrich, *Industrial Accident Prevention,* p. 427.
[5] Heinrich, *Industrial Accident Prevention,* p. 427.

In 1908 New York passed the first workmen's compensation law, which said, in effect, that regardless of fault, industry would pay for injuries occurring on the job. The law was later held unconstitutional. However, in 1911 Wisconsin passed similar legislation, and this time it was held constitutional.[6] The stage was now set for future workmen's compensation laws, which would provide much impetus for the beginning of the industrial safety movement.

Workmen's compensation laws gave the employer a direct financial interest in the accident problem. Today industry accepts almost without exception the idea of financial responsibility for work injuries.[7] After the passage of the early workmen's compensation laws, industry was forced to seek financial protection through insurance. This meant that they were rated for premium payments in accordance with their accident records. In the process of trying to save money on insurance premiums, industry discovered that safety programs increased production.

THE MODERN INDUSTRIAL SAFETY MOVEMENT

The modern industrial safety movement dates from about 1912. By this time several groups from industry, employee organizations, and insurance companies were expressing an interest in industrial safety. As a result, the National Council for Industrial Safety was formed in 1913. Due to its growth and extension into other areas of public safety, the name was changed in 1915 to the National Safety Council.[8] This organization has led all our major efforts in safety, and under its guidance, the accident rates in industry have been reduced dramatically in the last 60 years.

In 1931 H. W. Heinrich published a revolutionary book called *Industrial Accident Prevention*. It suggested that unsafe acts of people were the causes of a high percentage of accidents. The book became the blueprint for modern safety programs. Many of our programs today operate within the framework of Heinrich's theories.[9] As we know, until that time the primary emphasis had been on the removal of environmental hazards.

Just how effective the modern safety movement in industry has been is evidenced by the following facts. Between 1912 and 1972, accidental work deaths per 100,000 population were reduced from 21 to 7. In 1912 an estimated 18,000 to 21,000 lives were lost in work accidents. By 1972

[6] Petersen, *Techniques of Safety Management*, p. 10.
[7] National Safety Council, *Accident Prevention Manual for Industrial Operations*, 6th ed. (Chicago, 1969), p. 17.
[8] Heinrich, *Industrial Accident Prevention*, p. 429.
[9] Petersen, *Techniques of Safety Management*, p. 11.

this figure had been reduced to approximately 14,100. In the years between 1912 and 1972, the work force doubled in size, and production increased seven times.[10] Figure 6-1 illustrates the reduction in deaths and death rates that has occurred since 1935.

A closer examination of Figure 6-1 shows that since about 1954 the number of deaths from industrial accidents has been relatively stable. It is hard to believe that we have reached an irreducible minimum of occupational accidental deaths. What this does indicate is a need for thorough investigation into why this phenomenon has occurred. To reach a stalemate and at the same time to continue to lose 14,000 lives a year in industrial programs indicates a definite need for reevaluation of our present industrial safety techniques. (This stalemate, combined with weak state and federal occupational safety laws, instigated the birth of the Occupational Safety and Health Act of 1970.)

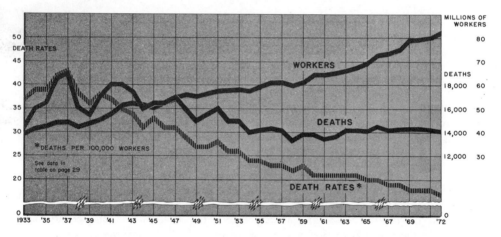

Figure 6-1. *Industrial deaths and death rate trends. Reproduced from* Accident Facts 1973 Edition, *p. 23, courtesy of the National Safety Council.*

Member companies of the National Safety Council generally have better safety programs than nonmember companies and they generally have lower injury rates.[11] Obviously safety programs *do* pay dividends. (See Tables 6-1 and 6-2.)

What are the causes of industrial accidents? Falls and handling of objects account for one-half of all temporary work injuries, according to state labor department reports. Machinery accidents account for 6 percent

[10] National Safety Council, *Accident Facts 1973 Edition* (Chicago, 1973), p. 23.

[11] National Safety Council, *Accident Facts 1973*, p. 27.

Table 6-1. Frequency rates, NSC members versus national experience, 1969-1971.

Industry (NSC Classification)	1969		1970		1971	
	NSC	BLS	NSC	BLS	NSC	BLS
Aerospace............................	2.4	4.3	2.8	4.5	2.3	...
Automobile...........................	1.7	6.1	1.5	5.3	1.4	...
Chemical.............................	4.0	7.8	4.3	8.3	4.8	...
Fertilizer.............................	6.2	12.6	5.7	11.9	7.5	...
Food.................................	13.1	24.2	14.6	25.4	15.1	...
Foundry..............................	12.4	30.5	13.6	33.7	12.3	...
Glass................................	7.8	11.0	8.5	13.8	9.1	...
Iron and Steel Products.................	11.4	21.3	11.3	23.2	11.1	...
Lumber..............................	15.4	36.4	14.6	37.2	13.9	...
Machinery............................	4.9	14.1	4.8	14.0	4.9	...
Mining, Coal..........................	29.7	43.3	32.4	42.5	34.6	45.9
Mining, Metal and Nonmetal..............	19.9	29.3	23.4	30.7	17.2	26.1
Non-ferrous Metals and Products.........	9.4	19.5	9.3	17.2	9.5	...
Pulp and Paper........................	8.9	16.2	8.4	13.9	8.5	...
Quarrying, Stone, Sand and Gravel.......	17.3	20.9	18.7	22.1	18.0	21.9
Rubber and Plastics....................	4.9	17.7	5.4	18.6	6.5	...
Sheet Metal Products..................	5.5	22.3	5.1	21.8	5.2	...
Steel.................................	3.5	7.3	3.4	6.5	3.6	...
Textile...............................	4.2	8.9	3.9	8.8	4.2	...
Wood Products........................	14.3	26.6	12.3	25.5	12.8	...

Source: NSC—reporters to National Safety Council, except Mining and Quarrying industries which are from U.S. Bureau of Mines safety competitions; BLS—reporters to U.S. Bureau of Labor Statistics, except for Mining and Quarrying industries which are industrywide data from Bureau of Mines.

Reproduced from Accident Facts 1973 Edition, *p. 27, courtesy of the National Safety Council.*

Table 6-2. Comparative injury rates—NSC members and nonmembers.

Year	Injury Frequency Rate			Injury Severity Rate		
	NSC Members	Non-members	% NSC Rates Lower	NSC Members	Non-members	% NSC Rates Lower
	Manufacturing					
1965..........	4.6	16.8	−73	450	830	−46
1966..........	5.1	17.6	−71	470	810	−42
1967..........	5.1	18.0	−72	460	830	−45
1968..........	5.3	17.9	−70	480	790	−39
1969..........	5.7	18.9	−70	500	830	−40
1970..........	6.0	19.1	−69	500	860	−42
1971..........	6.0	**	..	450	**	..
1972..........	6.3	**	..	470	**	..
	Mining					
1965..........	23.5	37.9	−38	4,024	6,970	−42
1966..........	21.9	38.4	−43	4,016	6,534	−39
1967..........	22.4	37.5	−40	4,019	6,092	−34
1968..........	22.2	36.7	−40	4,494	7,983	−44
1969..........	21.8	37.6	−42	3,597	6,506	−45
1970..........	22.2	39.2	−43	3,793	6,644	−43
1971..........	22.2	33.4	−34	3,277	4,260	−23

Source: Manufacturing nonmember—Total U. S. experience projected from BLS rates, less experience of reporters to NSC. Mining nonmember—Industrywide rates from Bureau of Mines, less reporters in U. S. Bureau of Mines safety competitions.   **Not available.

Reproduced from Accident Facts 1973 Edition, *p. 27, courtesy of the National Safety Council.*

of the total temporary injuries, 19 percent of the permanent partial in
juries, and 3 percent of the fatal injuries or permanent total disabilities.
Motor vehicle accidents account for 18 percent of the fatal and permanent

injury cases, but only 4 and 5 percent of the permanent partial and temporary total injuries. For all cases, motor vehicle injuries and falls are among the most costly.[12]

Work injuries occur most frequently in the first hour of the work day and least frequently in the fifth and ninth hours. The fifth hour usually follows lunch, and the ninth and later hours represent mostly overtime work. A rate based on exposure would be higher for overtime hours than for other hours of the work day.[13] Fatigue may be a factor.

Figure 6-2 classifies work accidents according to the part of the body that is most often injured. As you can see, injuries to the trunk occur most frequently.

Aside from the pain and anguish to the worker, industrial accidents cause a serious erosion in industrial profits. For example, Figure 6-3

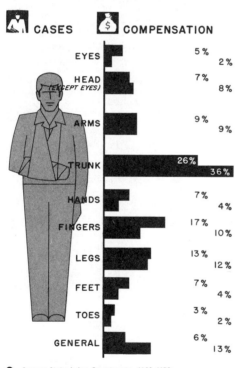

Disabling work injuries in the entire nation totalled approximately 2,400,000 in 1972. Of these, about 14,100 were fatal and 90,000 resulted in some permanent impairment.

Injuries to the trunk occurred most frequently, with thumb and finger injuries next, according to State Labor Department reports.

Eyes.....................120,000
Head (except eyes).......170,000
Arms....................220,000
Trunk..................630,000
Hands..................170,000
Fingers................400,000
Legs....................300,000
Feet....................170,000
Toes.................... 70,000
General................150,000

The chart shows for each body part, per cent of all injuries, and per cent of all compensation paid.

Source: State Labor Departments, 1969-1970; cases — 13 States, compensation — 8 States.

Figure 6-2. *Parts of the body injured in work accidents. Reproduced from* Accident Facts 1973 Edition, *p. 30, courtesy of the National Safety Council.*

[12] National Safety Council, *Accident Facts 1973*, p. 31.
[13] National Safety Council, *Accident Facts 1973*, p. 31.

TOTAL COST IN 1972 _____ $11,500,000,000*

   Visible Costs _____ 5,200,000,000

   Other Costs _____ 5,200,000,000

   Fire Losses _____ 1,100,000,000

   Cost Per Worker to Industry _____ 140

*Not included is the value of property damage in all accidents, except direct losses in fires.

Figure 6-3. *The cost of work accidents. Reproduced from* Accident Facts *1973 Edition, p. 24, courtesy of the National Safety Council.*

reveals an average cost of $140 per worker. This translates into a yearly cost of approximately $14,000,000 for an industry employing 10,000 workers.

Visible costs include wage losses, insurance, and administrative and medical costs. Other costs include the money value of time lost by workers (other than those with disabling injuries) who are directly or indirectly involved in accidents. This also includes the time required to investigate accidents and complete accident reports. Ironically, in today's modern society it is safer for the worker to be on than off the job. As Table 6-3 illustrates, "since World War II, accidental deaths of workers on the job have decreased by 15 per cent. Off the job, 1972 deaths exceeded the 1945

Table 6-3. *Trends in on-job and off-job deaths and injuries.*

Year	Deaths					Injuries		
	On–Job		Off–Job		Ratio Off/On	On-Job	Off-Job	Ratio Off/On
	No.	Rate*	No.	Rate*				
1945.........	16,500	33	30,000	60	1.82	2,000,000	2,750,000	1.38
1950.........	15,500	27	31,500	56	2.03	1,950,000	2,500,000	1.28
1955.........	14,200	24	31,300	53	2.20	1,950,000	2,400,000	1.23
1956.........	14,300	23	31,700	52	2.22	1,950,000	2,500,000	1.28
1957.........	14,200	23	31,700	52	2.23	1,900,000	2,450,000	1.29
1958.........	13,300	22	29,000	48	2.18	1,800,000	2,250,000	1.25
1959.........	13,800	23	29,000	47	2.10	1,950,000	2,200,000	1.13
1960.........	13,800	22	29,200	47	2.12	1,950,000	2,250,000	1.15
1961.........	13,500	21	28,900	45	2.14	1,950,000	2,200,000	1.16
1962.........	13,700	21	30,000	46	2.19	2,000,000	2,250,000	1.13
1963.........	14,200	21	31,700	48	2.23	2,000,000	2,350,000	1.18
1964.........	14,200	21	34,600	51	2.44	2,050,000	2,500,000	1.22
1965.........	14,100	20	36,500	52	2.59	2,100,000	2,700,000	1.29
1966.........	14,500	20	39,600	55	2.73	2,200,000	2,900,000	1.32
1967.........	14,200	19	40,000	54	2.82	2,200,000	3,000,000	1.36
1968.........	14,300	19	41,900	54	2.93	2,200,000	3,100,000	1.41
1969.........	14,300	18	43,300	55	3.03	2,200,000	3,200,000	1.45
1970.........	14,300	18	43,000	54	3.01	2,200,000	3,250,000	1.48
1971.........	14,200	18	41,500	52	2.92	2,300,000	3,200,000	1.39
1972.........	14,100	17	43,100	52	3.06	2,400,000	3,200,000	1.33
Change 1945-72.......	−15%	−48%	+44%	−13%	+68%	+20%	+16%	−4%

*Deaths per 100,000 workers.

Reproduced from Accident Facts 1973 Edition, *p. 25, courtesy of the National Safety Council.*

total by 44 per cent, but with an increase in the number of workers the *rate* was down 13 per cent. The ratio of off-job deaths to on-job deaths in 1972 was 3.06 to 1." [14]

FEDERAL LEGISLATION AFFECTING INDUSTRIAL SAFETY

Through the years several important federal laws have been enacted. The Social Security Act of 1935 provided workers with help for various kinds of economic setbacks. It also gave them a federal pension plan. The National Labor Relations Act of 1935 gave protection to the organizing rights of the worker, and this in turn raised safety standards. The Fair Labor Standards Act of 1938 contained provisions to prevent abuses in hours, wages, and work conditions.

In 1970 Congress passed the Occupational Safety and Health Act (OSHA). From the standpoint of worker health and safety, this law has the most far-reaching effects of any legislation in modern history. It applies to any business affecting interstate commerce, which means that virtually all businesses, regardless of size, are covered.

OSHA calls for all employers to comply with occupational safety and health standards promulgated under the act, and in addition employers must provide each of their employees with a place of employment free from recognized hazards that are causing or are likely to cause death or serious injury.[15]

In regard to the OSHA legislation, the National Safety Council says:

Standards are the very heart of the safety process established by the OSHAct. The safety and health standards promulgated by the Secretary of Labor are designed to protect working people from occupational injury and illness. These standards are the principal criteria which are used by OSHA compliance officers when inspecting establishments.
Safety and health standards are not an invention of the federal government. On the contrary, most of the OSHAct standards were developed by nationally recognized standards-producing organizations established mainly by and for industrial management.[16]

In addition to meeting the standards prescribed by the Secretary of Labor under the act, employers must notify employees of their protections

---

[14] National Safety Council, *Accident Facts 1973*, p. 25.
[15] "What Are the Provisions of the New Safety Act?" *Safety Standards*, March-April 1971, p. 5.
[16] National Safety Council, "OHSAct Primer, Part II: Standards," *National Safety News*, February 1973, p. 48.

and obligations under the law. Records must be kept of work-related deaths, illnesses, and injuries, as well as of employee exposure to potentially toxic materials and harmful physical agents. Employees must be notified of exposure to toxic material or harmful physical agents that exceed limits set forth in the standards.[17]

In addition, the Secretary has the authority to inspect and investigate any covered workplace. He also has the power to subpoena evidence in connection with the investigation.[18] Representatives of the employer and employee will be allowed to accompany the inspector on his visits. The employer or an employee can also request an inspection.

Several other provisions cover violations of the act with rather stringent penalties. The bill is largely effective because of these inspection and penalty provisions.

PROGRAMMING FOR INDUSTRIAL SAFETY

The purpose of programming for industrial safety is to promote safe and efficient production. Without doubt, accident reduction invariably leads to more efficient production, a fact oftentimes not well recognized by top management. The word "programming" suggests planning. Good safety programming does require both planning and execution. This means it must have management approval to be successful.

A prime example of a well-planned and well-executed industrial safety program is that of E. I. Du Pont De Nemours and Company, which holds an outstanding long-term performance record in accident prevention. In 1912, the first year that Du Pont kept injury records on a basis comparable to that now recommended by the National Safety Council, there were 43 lost-time injuries per million man-hours worked. Fifteen years later the number had dropped to 10 lost-time injuries per million man-hours worked. In 1931 the rate was 1.82. By 1969 it was 0.40, and by 1970 it had been reduced to 0.37.[19]

The cost of the 85 lost-time or permanent disabling injuries among the 100,000 Du Pont employees was an estimated $850,000 in 1969. Projected on the same ratio of all industry, which was 14.8 injuries per million man-hours, the cost would have been $30,000,000.[20] This is direct evidence that safety pays.

As we have said, one of the newer concepts in safety management is

[17] "What Are the Provisions of the New Safety Act?" p. 8.
[18] "What Are the Provisions of the New Safety Act?" p. 9.
[19] National Safety Council, "Preventing Accidents Pays Off," *National Safety News*, August 1971, p. 52.
[20] National Safety Council, "Preventing Accidents Pays Off," p. 52.

systems engineering for safety. A system is defined as simply an assemblage of things and parts that go together to make up a whole.[21] Systems safety considers man, machines, and the environment interacting together. John Flaherty says that man may select, alter, or partially control his environment, but he can never abandon it. Machines, he says, are actually extensions of man, and as such they come under his control and respond to his decisions.[22]

If we are to reduce accidents to an irreducible minimum, we must consider the whole system as it relates to the causes of those accidents. An accident is the result of some malfunction in that system which must be identified and corrected.

PRINCIPLES OF ACCIDENT PREVENTION

Dan Petersen lists the following principles for accident prevention:

1. An unsafe act, an unsafe condition, an accident: all these are symptoms of something wrong in the management system.
2. Certain sets of circumstances can be predicted to produce severe injuries. These circumstances can be identified and controlled.
3. Safety should be managed like any other company function. Management should direct the safety effort by setting achievable goals, by planning, organizing, and controlling to achieve them.
4. The key to effective line safety performance is management procedures that fix accountability.
5. The function of safety is to locate and define the operational errors that allow accidents to occur. This function can be carried out in two ways: (1) by asking why—searching for root causes of accidents; and (2) by asking whether or not certain known effective controls are being utilized.[23]

(See the section on "The Scope and Function of the Professional Safety Position" in Chapter 14.)

COMPONENTS OF AN INDUSTRIAL SAFETY PROGRAM

A modern industrial safety program consists of the following distinct components:

[21] W. C. Pope, "Safety and Systems Management," *National Safety News,* May 1971, p. 56.

[22] John Flaherty, "Systems Approach to Safety Supervision," *National Safety News,* February 1973, p. 52.

[23] Petersen, *Techniques of Safety Management,* pp. 19–22.

1. Complete management backing and leadership, with achievable goals determined.
2. Adequate records of accidents and injuries.
3. Detailed analysis of all accidents for the purposes of prevention.
4. Provision for mechanical safeguards.
5. Detailed task analysis of all the various jobs.
6. Development of safety rules based on past accident records and job analysis.
7. Training education procedures based on task analysis of the job and on safety requirements.
8. Evaluation of the safety programs.

complete management support

Management must place safety on a level of importance with quantity and quality of production and cost control. This involves the assignment of responsibility, with the ensuing accountability for the success or failure of the system.

adequate accident records

The primary purpose of accident records is to prevent the repetition of similar occurrences. Adequate records will provide a history of accidents, with frequency, severity, location, and other details. These records must meet the standards approved by the Occupational Safety and Health Act. If possible they should be in sufficient detail to provide design engineers with the necessary information for such things as upgrading safeguards on dangerous machinery. They should contain cost factors to help determine the dollar cost effectiveness of accident programs.

Adequate records are necessary to any meaningful program in accident prevention. Failure to fill out an accident investigation report constitutes a negligent act. Figure 6-4 illustrates a form acceptable for OSHA standards; a more detailed form would be preferred for engineering purposes.

analysis of accidents

The analysis of an accident should first determine the contributing causes. What were the immediate causes? Was it an unsafe act on the part of the victim or some other person? Was fatigue a factor? What was the person's mental condition at the time of the accident? Were safety rules being followed at the time? If not, why not? Were the safety rules adequate? What new training procedures or other preventative measures

OSHA No. 101
Case or File No. _____

Form approved
OMB No. 44R 1453

Supplementary Record of Occupational Injuries and Illnesses

EMPLOYER

1. Name _____

2. Mail address _____
          (No. and street)   (City or town)   (State)

3. Location, if different from mail address _____

INJURED OR ILL EMPLOYEE

4. Name _____ Social Security No. _____
      (First name)   (Middle name)   (Last name)

5. Home address _____
             (No. and street)   (City or town)   (State)

6. Age _____   7. Sex: Male_____ Female_____ (Check one)

8. Occupation _____
          (Enter regular job title, *not* the specific activity he was performing at time of injury.)

9. Department _____
          (Enter name of department or division in which the injured person is regularly employed, even
          though he may have been temporarily working in another department at the time of injury.)

THE ACCIDENT OR EXPOSURE TO OCCUPATIONAL ILLNESS

10. Place of accident or exposure _____
              (No. and street)   (City or town)   (State)
    If accident or exposure occurred on employer's premises, give address of plant or establishment in which
    it occurred. Do not indicate department or division within the plant or establishment. If accident oc-
    curred outside employer's premises at an identifiable address, give that address. If it occurred on a pub-
    lic highway or at any other place which cannot be identified by number and street, please provide place
    references locating the place of injury as accurately as possible.

11. Was place of accident or exposure on employer's premises? _____ (Yes or No)

12. What was the employee doing when injured? _____
                                  (Be specific. If he was using tools or equipment or handling material,
    _____
                        name them and tell what he was doing with them.)

13. How did the accident occur? _____
                              (Describe fully the events which resulted in the injury or occupational illness. Tell what
    _____
    happened and how it happened. Name any objects or substances involved and tell how they were involved. Give
    _____
    full details on all factors which led or contributed to the accident. Use separate sheet for additional space.)

OCCUPATIONAL INJURY OR OCCUPATIONAL ILLNESS

14. Describe the injury or illness in detail and indicate the part of body affected. _____
                                                  (e.g.: amputation of right index finger
    _____
          at second joint; fracture of ribs; lead poisoning; dermatitis of left hand, etc.)

15. Name the object or substance which directly injured the employee. (For example, the machine or thing
    he struck against or which struck him; the vapor or poison he inhaled or swallowed; the chemical or ra-
    diation which irritated his skin; or in cases of strains, hernias, etc., the thing he was lifting, pulling, etc.)
    _____
    _____

16. Date of injury or initial diagnosis of occupational illness _____
                                                        (Date)

17. Did employee die? _____ (Yes or No)

OTHER

18. Name and address of physician _____

19. If hospitalized, name and address of hospital _____
    _____

    Date of report _____ **Prepared by** _____
    Official position _____

Figure 6-4. An OSHA-approved accident form. Courtesy of the National Safety Council.

could be utilized to prevent the accident from repeating itself? Obviously this requires evaluation of the entire system to determine the root causes of accidents.

The four principal methods of analysis of accidents are: failure mode and effect; fault tree; THERP (technique for human error prediction); and cost effectiveness. These methods each have variations, and they may be combined in a single analysis.[24] A detailed description of these methods can be found in industrial safety manuals. Also see the section on Systems Safety Analysis in Chapter 3.

provision for mechanical safeguards

Provision for mechanical safeguards represents one of the earliest efforts in industrial safety programs. Today, with systems engineering techniques, this has become very sophisticated. Every effort should be exerted to make certain that built-in safety precautions accompany all equipment. Human variables and the possibility for human error should be considered in the early design of all equipment and machinery. When feasible, the equipment should be rendered inoperable when the mechanical safeguards are not properly in place. Figure 6-5 illustrates some mechanical safeguards presently in use in industry, and also some protective equipment.

task analysis of the job

A detailed task analysis of a specific job will show what is involved in performing it. It should reveal what training procedures are necessary and what approaches can make those training procedures meaningful to the employee. Figure 6-6 illustrates what might be involved in a task analysis of a specific job.

This approach takes into account the necessity for individualized employee training. Russell DeReamer suggests the following key elements in job hazard analysis.[25]

1. Job description.
2. Job location.
3. Key job steps.
4. Tools used.

---

[24] J. T. Becht, *Systems Safety Analysis: A Modern Approach to Safety Problems*, special publication (Chicago: The National Safety Council, n.d.), p. 3.

[25] Russell DeReamer, *Modern Safety Practices* (New York: John Wiley & Sons, 1958), p. 49.

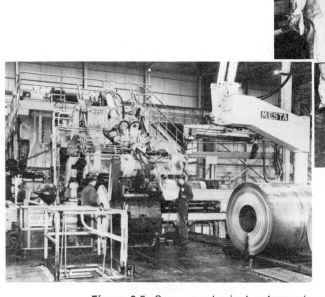

Figure 6-5. *Some mechanical safeguards and protective devices used in industry. Courtesy of United States Steel Corporation, Gary Works, Gary, Indiana.*

5. Potential health and injury hazards.
6. Safe practices, apparel, and equipment.

development of safety rules

Safety rules should be developed as a cooperative effort, with the individual employee playing a key part. His participation is vital if the rules are to be followed. Safety rules must be meaningful and strictly enforced for the good of all employees. This is one area in which both management and labor come to agreement. Both individual and mass training sessions should emphasize these rules, and it should be clearly understood that they are to be followed at all times. Failure to follow established safety rules should be grounds for dismissal. Also, manage-

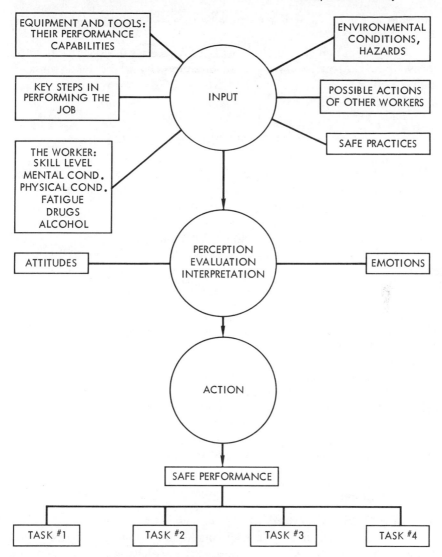

Figure 6-6. *A task analysis of a job.*

ment should be held accountable for development of the rules and the training sessions to implement them.

evaluation of the safety program

Continuous and ongoing evaluation is a necessary element of any industrial safety program. Various methods and formulas are available, and most of them take into account such things as severity and frequency of accidents.

The evaluation should show where the failures are occurring within the system. Corrective or remedial measures should be taken immediately.

COMMON HEALTH HAZARDS IN INDUSTRY

The modern safety professional in industry is no longer interested in only those events or accidents that cause immediate injury or death. He is also highly concerned with those conditions that encourage the development of the slow, insidious diseases which affect various parts of the body, such as the lungs, skin, kidneys, or brain.[26]

The science that deals with these conditions is known as Industrial Hygiene, defined as:

> That science (or art) devoted to the recognition, evaluation, and control of those environmental factors or stresses, chemical, physical, biological, and ergonomic, that may cause sickness, impaired health, or significant discomfort to employees or residents of the community.[27]

The industrial hygienist works closely with the safety professional and medical departments in modern industry. Since the safety professional is interested in day-to-day safety functions, he must know when and where to go for help on problems involving industrial hygiene.[28] Therefore the work and presence of an industrial hygienist can be of considerable importance to the health of employees.

chemical hazards

Chemicals—in the form of vapors, gases, dusts, fumes, and mists—represent the major health hazard among many industrial operations. These agents enter the body in various ways, such as inhalation, ingestion through the mouth, and skin absorption. In order to be harmful they must come in contact with a body cell.[29]

The method of entry becomes important because it will determine

---

[26] National Safety Council, *Fundamentals of Industrial Hygiene* (Chicago, 1971), p. 1.
[27] National Safety Council, *Fundamentals of Industrial Hygiene*, p. 1.
[28] National Safety Council, *Fundamentals of Industrial Hygiene*, p. 5.
[29] National Safety Council, *Fundamentals of Industrial Hygiene*, p. 5.

what control can be used to eliminate the hazard. Some of the agents, such as TNT and the cyanides, can cause systemic poisoning after direct contact with the skin.[30] Many agents cause skin irritation. Inhaling chemicals is dangerous because of the rapidity with which they can be absorbed by the lungs and then passed into the bloodstream, and on to the brain. This same material, if ingested, would be considerably diluted because of the contents in the stomach.[31] However, many potentially harmful chemical agents are ingested through the mouth.

Obviously it is important that the safety professional have a thorough knowledge of the chemicals being utilized both in the manufacturing process and in the final product. The large number of chemical agents four 1 in industrial operations, their ability to enter the human body in various ways, and the high sensitivity of the human being to these agents make them an extremely important factor in the health of employees.

Some chemicals are especially dangerous because of factors such as flammability or instability. The safety person and the employees must be fully aware of these hazards.

physical health hazards

The physical health hazards common to industrial operations are usually found in the form of: [32]

1. Extremes of temperature.
2. Extremes of pressure.
3. Mechanical vibration and repeated motion.
4. Radiation.
5. Noise.

These have both immediate and cumulative effects on the worker. They should be just as important to the safety worker as are the other types of health hazards.

Heat exhaustion, heat stroke, and frozen limbs may result from extreme temperature exposures. The bends, caused by formation of nitrogen bubbles in the blood, are the result of rapid decompression. Air hammers, stone cutting tools, and other equipment cause damage from vibration, and there are several forms of harmful radiation. Some for-

---

[30] National Safety Council, *Fundamentals of Industrial Hygiene*, p. 7.
[31] National Safety Council, *Fundamentals of Industrial Hygiene*, p. 7.
[32] National Safety Council, *Fundamentals of Industrial Hygiene*, p. 25.

ward-looking industries carry on rather extensive hearing conservation programs, where noise is considered a harmful factor.

biological health hazards

Biological health hazards in industry usually take the form of some disease caused by a specific agent related to that industry. For example, tuberculosis may be contracted by nurses, doctors, or attendants caring for tuberculosis patients. Workers exposed to various kinds of dust are subject to upper respiratory infections. For example, dusts from vegetable fibers such as cotton, hemp, flax, or grain may cause problems ranging from chronic irritation of the nose and throat to bronchitis, complicated by asthma, emphysema, or pneumonia.

SUMMARY

The industrial safety picture is the "bright spot" in the entire accident prevention movement, for it represents the area of greatest improvement. However, industrial safety has probably received more emphasis over a longer period of time than any other safety area. Definite progressive and influential steps can be traced through the history of industrial safety. The first laws called for inspection and regulation; they were followed by workmen's compensation laws that forced industry to become active in the movement. Heinrich's work in 1931 shifted the emphasis to human error as well as environmental control, a shift that had dramatic effects on industrial safety. Today systems engineering will undoubtedly prove beneficial. The Occupational Safety and Health Act should upgrade all safety standards, especially in the smaller industries and in the larger industries exhibiting poor safety records.

In the final analysis, those forward-looking companies that have achieved such outstanding safety records in comparison to others did so not by luck but through planning and execution of good safety programs. It required the expenditure of huge sums of money and a conviction that this was the right thing to do. The by-product for the companies was not only the satisfaction of saving lives and reducing pain and misery, but also the amount of money saved as well as bigger profits earned.

Safety programs contribute immeasurably to the morale of any company. They foster a spirit of team play and decorum that can only result in pride felt by management and employees alike. The end result is safe and efficient production. Safety programs should rank in importance with the amount, quality, and cost of production.

SUGGESTED STUDENT ACTIVITIES

1. Make a task analysis diagram of a particular job that you perform regularly.
2. Visit the safety director on your campus, if possible, and try to reconstruct an actual accident to determine possible causes.
3. Visit the director of safety of an industrial plant and ascertain the different phases in its safety program.
4. Develop plans for a mass safety education program for an industrial plant in your area.
5. Write a report on "black lung" disease.
6. Visit your nearest OSHA district office and find out which industries in your area have the best, and which the poorest, accident records.
7. Write a report on systems engineering. Research the four methods of accident analysis.
8. Write a task analysis of an industrial hygienist, with suggested course work to qualify for the job.
9. Keep a record for one month of all occupational hazards in the places you normally visit, such as grocery stores and service stations.
10. Invite a safety supervisor or OSHA inspector to speak before your class or group.

BIBLIOGRAPHY

DeReamer, Russell. *Modern Safety Practices.* New York: John Wiley & Sons, 1958.

Flaherty, John. "Systems Approach to Safety Supervision." *National Safety News,* February 1973, p. 52.

Heinrich, H. W. *Industrial Accident Prevention.* New York: McGraw-Hill Book Co., 1959.

National Safety Council. *Accident Facts 1973 Edition.* Chicago, 1973.

————. *Accident Prevention Manual for Industrial Operations.* 6th ed. Chicago, 1969.

————. *Fundamentals of Industrial Hygiene.* Chicago, 1971.

————. "OSHAct Primer, Part II: Standards." *National Safety News,* February 1973, p. 48.

————. "Preventing Accidents Pays Off." *National Safety News,* August 1971, p. 52.

Petersen, Dan. *Techniques of Safety Management.* New York: McGraw-Hill Book Co., 1971.

Pope, W. C. "Safety and Systems Management." *National Safety News,* May 1971, p. 56.

Recht, J. L. *Systems Safety Analysis: A Modern Approach to Safety Problems.* Special publication. Chicago: The National Safety Council, n.d.

Simonds, R. H., and Grimaldi, J. V. *Safety Management.* Homewood, Ill.: Richard D. Irwin, Inc., 1963.

"What Are the Provisions of the New Safety Act?" *Safety Standards,* March–April 1971.

7

farm safety

Modern agriculture, the most basic industry in the world, has entered the systems era. Versatile hydraulic systems give tractor operators control over their work. Computerized systems offer milk producers print-out readings of the intake-output ratio of dairy cows, and automatic feeding systems control the amount of grain fed to livestock.[1] Automated equipment allows the farmer to produce crops virtually without ever touching the seed or the final product by hand.

Figure 7-1 shows what a typical American farm may look like in the year 2000. Note in the right background a high-rise cattle barn, with a completely controlled environment. In the left background is a warehouse complex and refinery where waste from the barn will be purified and recirculated to the barn. At the right is a huge plastic dome covering ten or more acres, where crops will be grown in a computer-controlled environment for maximum production. To the left of the dome is a farmhouse, and in front of it the control center from which the farmer will direct an array of equipment and personnel by electronic machines that are just now being developed.

[1] National Safety Council, *Farm and Ranch Safety Guide* (Chicago, 1973), p. 5.

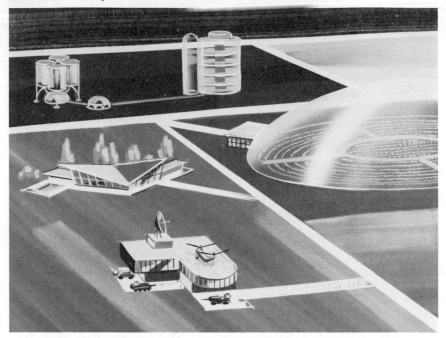

Figure 7-1. A farm will probably look like this in the year 2000. Courtesy of Ford Motor Company, Tractor Operations.

THE PRESENT STATUS OF FARM
SAFETY PROGRAMS

Modern technology has provided the basis for a great revolution in farming operations, and will continue to do so. The small farm is gradually disappearing and being replaced by larger, modernized farms with production methods undreamed of a few years ago. Along with the increase in size of individual farming operations has come a decrease in the number of people actively engaged in farming. It is estimated that only about 4 percent of the gainfully employed people in the United States today are engaged in farming, compared to approximately 14 percent in 1947. Despite a reduction in the number of workers, production has increased tremendously. If it had not, the problems of world food supply would be insurmountable.

Modern machinery and better understanding of the techniques of crop production have revolutionized agriculture. Most of this technology has come about in the last few years, bringing with it a multitude of new hazards, perhaps larger in variety than that experienced by most industries.

Today's farmer must work with automated equipment, some of which can start up unexpectedly. He must deal with improved technology in chemicals, and he is also subject to animal-related diseases and injuries. Add to these the unique hazards of the farm environment, such as weather, excessive dust, poisonous and toxic gases, inflammable liquids, and others, and you can begin to see the tremendous safety problems peculiar to the agriculture industry.

Other problems unique to farming increase the risk of accidents. The farmer must be most productive during a limited number of days when the weather and climatic conditions are favorable to his crops. Therefore he must work long hours under fatigue in many cases. He is often faced with a multifaceted type of production. Many modern farms simultaneously produce grain crops, livestock, and a host of dairy products. The farmer must be a manager, a supervisor, a worker, a mechanic, a safety engineer, and many other things to be successful and safe.

One result of these farming safety problems is 2,200 accidental work deaths per year.[2] They are part of the total 14,100 occupational deaths per year in all industries. The 2,200 deaths represent an accidental death rate of 61 per 100,000 agricultural workers, compared to a combined rate of 17 for all industries.[3] The accidental death rate in agriculture is exceeded only by the accidental death rates in mining and construction. To these 2,200 accidental deaths per year are added about 200,000 work-related disabling injuries.[4]

The immediate problem is to reduce these unduly high accident rates in agriculture. Over the years several groups have been interested in doing just that. Some have made extensive contributions despite the major stumbling block of insufficient accident data. The National Safety Council has long been a leader in agricultural accident prevention. It recognizes the lack of accident data and has consistently pushed for more adequate collection methods. The Occupational Safety and Health Act will mean stronger federal intervention into agricultural safety.

Why is the lack of adequate accident data such a stumbling block in the prevention of accidents in agriculture? Accident data analysis allows safety professionals to determine more specific proximate and contributing causes of farm accidents. It would allow agricultural engineers and educators to assign priorities. Farm equipment manufacturers could make better use of human factors engineering in the upgrading of their equipment.

Accident analysis would provide the basis for other systems engineering techniques, such as the task analysis approach to farm jobs. As

[2] National Safety Council, *Accident Facts 1973 Edition* (Chicago, 1973), p. 85.
[3] National Safety Council, *Accident Facts 1973*, p. 23.
[4] National Safety Council, *Accident Facts 1973*, p. 23.

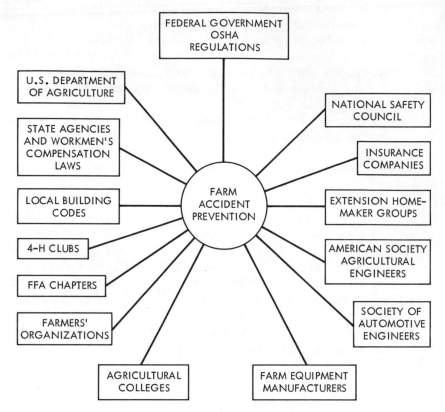

Figure 7-2. *Organizations interested in agricultural safety.*

with other industries, task analysis can give answers to the methods and emphasis needed for training programs. Adequate accident data with proper analysis would provide the basis for a coordinated and meaningful approach to farm accident reduction efforts.

Why is there such a glaring deficiency in present accident data concerning agricultural operations? What is being done about the problem? Agricultural operations are not united. The agricultural industry is a collection of millions of people working separately or in small groups, as compared to most industries where there are hundreds or even thousands working under one roof and under controlled and supervised conditions.

Accident data collection has been fragmentary as a result of these segregated operations. Since agricultural workers are not concentrated, the accidents, even if reported, also lack concentration. Therefore they

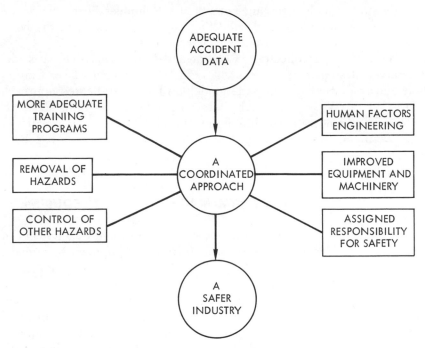

Figure 7-3. Farm accident prevention programming.

do not get sufficient attention to arouse public concern. The isolation of agricultural operations has also made the process of collecting accident data both difficult and unduly expensive.

Research into farm work accidents has generally been in the form of scattered studies on a county or state basis, usually originating in universities. Until recently only a few studies of areas containing large numbers of farmers have been completed. However, in 1971 Michigan State University completed a study of exposure to farm machinery in Michigan and Ohio. Random stratified sampling techniques were employed, and the study covered approximately 2,200 farms.[5] The Michigan–Ohio study gave consideration to "exposure"; thus accident frequency rates were established.

Under the leadership of the National Safety Council, surveys of even larger scope are underway. They should eventually turn into na-

[5] Howard J. Doss and Richard G. Pfister, *Nature and Extent of Farm Machinery Use in Relation to Frequency of Accidents,* Agricultural Engineering Department, Center for Rural Manpower and Public Affairs, Report No. 30 (East Lansing, Michigan: Michigan State University, 1971), pp. 1, 6.

tionwide studies with recurring potentiality. Volunteer farm groups are conducting the interviews and collecting the data, overcoming the heretofore prohibitive cost and isolation factors.

Thus, with the collection of accident data on a massive basis, the necessary first step in farm accident reduction is taking place. Careful study and analysis should provide guidelines for a coordinated approach to farm safety. We can reasonably expect a reduction in farm accidents and farm accident rates within a few years. This reduction will not come overnight, but the picture certainly is the brightest it has been for years.

MAN, FARM MACHINERY, AND EQUIPMENT

Farm machinery and equipment account for approximately 20 percent of all farm work accidents. Yet, farm machinery and equipment have made possible the transition from small to large farm operations, at the same time using fewer people with resulting increases in production.

Farming is a perfect example of the interaction between man, machines, and environment. Complicated farm machinery is being operated by man in an environment with special problems of weather, temperature, visibility, atmospheric pollution, and so forth.[6] It is usually a malfunction in this interaction process that causes an accident. The human element is the biggest single contributing factor. It includes such things such as illness, alcohol, poor vision, age, inexperience, poor attitudes, and ignorance of safety rules. The opportunity for human error is increased in farming operations because of certain job-related factors— distraction resulting from long, jolting, monotonous hours on tractors or the effects of heat, cold, wind, rain, dust, and excessive noise.[7] Lack of proper protective equipment and mechanical malfunctions are other contributing factors to human error.[8]

Since human error is the major factor in all accidents, it is not surprising that farm accident rates are high, for there are many job-related factors on the farm that can generate even more human error. The extent to which the farmer recognizes and compensates for the extra hazards inherent in farming will determine to a large extent how safe he is.

The tractor is the most essential part of today's modern farm equipment. It is also responsible for 800 to 1,000 of the 2,200 farm work fatali-

[6] National Safety Council, *Safe Tractor Operation*, Rural Accident Prevention Bulletin (Chicago, n.d.), p. 1.
[7] National Safety Council, *Safe Tractor Operation*, p. 2.
[8] National Safety Council, *Safe Tractor Operation*, p. 2.

ties per year, as well as for tens of thousands of work-related disabling injuries.[9]

More than one-half of the tractor accident fatalities result from overturn, which causes many serious injuries and expensive property damage as well. Tractor overturns are usually caused by such things as driving too fast for conditions, working on steep slopes, striking surface hazards, hitching loads too high, and improperly operating front end loaders.[10]

Roll-over bars and protective cabs are effective in preventing death and injury. Today's required use of seat belts with roll-over bars and cabs should further reduce injuries and deaths.

Other common causes of tractor mishaps are:

1. Falling from the tractor.
2. Being caught in the power takeoff shaft or joint.
3. Running into or over a bystander or another worker.
4. Striking overhead hazards.
5. Colliding with a motor vehicle or roadside object.
6. Being struck by flying objects.
7. Being fallen on by a poorly supported tractor while performing maintenance.
8. Being overcome by fumes inside a building.
9. Sustaining cuts, bruises, or burns during maintenance operations.
10. Sustaining burns during fueling operations or tractor fires.[11]

The Michigan–Ohio study indicated that tractor operations have high accident frequency rates on public roads and highways, as compared to general farm or tractor work. The study showed high accident rates especially for operators under 15 years of age and those 65 and older. This became very significant when operators in these age groups used tractors on public highways.[12]

The mechanization of pull-type equipment resulted in the use of a power transfer system called the power takeoff on tractors. There have been many improvements in the power takeoff systems in recent years, and the newer versions are completely shielded. However, if the farmer removes the shield for some purpose such as repairs and then fails to replace it, all the protection is lost.

[9] National Safety Council, *Safe Tractor Operation*, p. 1.
[10] National Safety Council, *Safe Tractor Operation*, p. 1.
[11] National Safety Council, *Safe Tractor Operation*, p. 1.
[12] Doss and Pfister, *Farm Machinery Use*, p. 21.

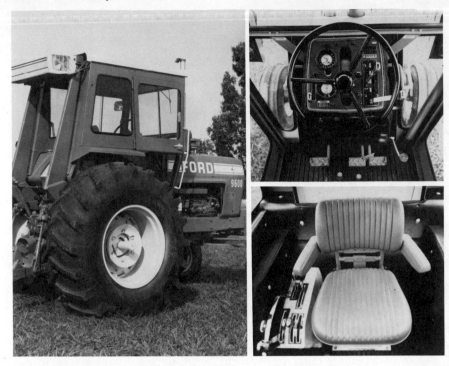

Figure 7-4. A tractor with a protective roll-over cab. Cabs of this type are often pressurized and air-conditioned. Photo courtesy of Ford Motor Company, Tractor Operations.

Many of the new tractors operating on farms have air-conditioned, fully pressurized cabs that give maximum protection against such factors as dust. Almost all tractor manufacturers offer these features today, adding much to the operator's safety, comfort, and convenience.

Some suggested measures to prevent tractor accidents are:

1. More emphasis on tractor training operations for pre-high school workers (15 and under). 4-H Clubs should expand their activities in this area.[13]
2. Increased safety programs for operators of all age groups by various farmer organizations.
3. More emphasis by high school driver education classes on prevention of collisions with all slow-moving vehicles.[14]
4. Use of the mass media to educate the public to the problem.[15]

[13] Doss and Pfister, *Farm Machinery Use*, p. 23.
[14] Doss and Pfister, *Farm Machinery Use*, p. 23.
[15] Doss and Pfister, *Farm Machinery Use*, p. 23.

Special emphasis should be given to slow-moving vehicles during the months when tractor accidents are frequent on public roadways.

5. Stricter enforcement of regulations requiring the use and maintenance of emblems that identify slow-moving vehicles. This emblem is a triangle with a fluorescent yellow-orange center for daylight visibility and a red reflective border for night.

6. Legislation requiring adequate roll-over protection.

7. Legislation making certain safety devices such as headlights, tail lights, and mirrors mandatory equipment on all tractors.

8. Increased emphasis by the manufacturers on the production of a more stable tractor.

9. More emphasis on the use of personal protective equipment such as hard hats, safety glasses, and fire extinguishers.

Another source of many farm injuries and deaths are portable augers and elevators, found on many farms that grow corn, beans, small grain, and hay. They are used for moving materials into bins, cribs, mows, or other storage facilities.[16] Injuries related to elevators and augers range from lacerations and fractures to amputations and even death.

Although this equipment actually has few moving parts, the opportunity for exposure is great, particularly to the conveying mechanism such as augers and elevator flights. The material to be conveyed must have access to the conveyor mechanism; thus the operator also is exposed to contact with the auger or elevator flight. Most of these accidents happen in the later afternoon during the harvest season.[17]

Today's modern combines, although supposedly safer than the old corn pickers, are still a source of accidents. Combines pull stalks through at a speed of nearly 20 feet per second. Human reaction time is three-quarters of a second. Therefore if a person was trying to unclog one of these machines and had taken hold of a cornstalk, only to have the machine suddenly jerk on the stalk, it could pull 15 feet of stalk through before the person could react and release the stalk.[18] Unclogging operations should therefore take place only after the machinery is completely shut down.

More progressive farmers today are making use of the task analysis approach to different farm jobs. This innovation into farming will provide the basis for better on-the-job training methods, which should reduce accidents. Figure 7-5 shows a sample task analysis.

[16] William J. Fletcher, "Avoiding Elevator and Auger Accidents," *Farm Safety Review*, November-December 1969, p. 5.

[17] Fletcher, "Avoiding Elevator and Auger Accidents," p. 5.

[18] Fletcher, "Avoiding Elevator and Auger Accidents," p. 6.

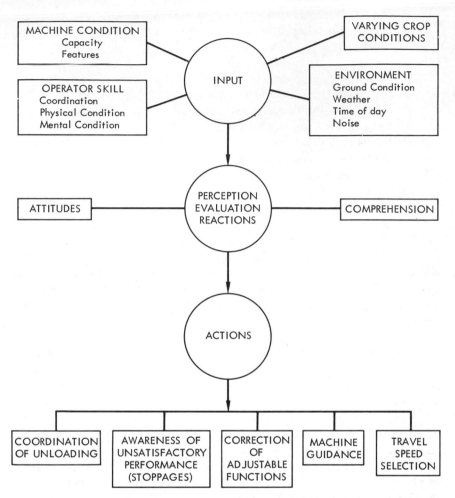

Figure 7-5. *Analysis of the combine operation process. Prepared by William Fletcher and William Hanford, Agricultural Engineers, National Safety Council.*

Wagons are almost as common as tractors on today's farms, according to a survey by the National Safety Council. They also produce a high number of injuries. Being caught "in between" and falling are common occurrences with wagons.[19]

The list of farm equipment and machinery in use today is extensive and may range from very heavy machinery to light power hand-held tools. This adds to the hazards on farms. In most industrial operations

[19] National Safety Council, "Ten State Accident Survey," *Farm Safety Review,* May-June 1973, p. 9.

the individual worker does not operate many types of equipment—he is more specialized than the farmer. The lack of specialization of farmers and the necessity for handling many kinds of equipment are undoubtedly a contributing factor in some farm accidents.

LIVESTOCK SAFETY

Farms contain many different kinds of animals, each with special characteristics and different ways of being hazardous. Most of the dangers in handling livestock can be eliminated by exercising proper safety precautions. Livestock safety programs have two primary concerns:

1. Prevention of accidents caused by improper handling of livestock.
2. Prevention of diseases that are transmitted from animal to man.

Even though accidents involving livestock have been reduced in recent years, they are still a major source of farm injuries and deaths every year. Successful livestock safety programs are based on good farm conditions—well-arranged feed lots, adequate facilities for sorting, penning, loading, and more.

milk cows

Milk cows cause more farm accidents than any other farm animals. Approximately two thirds of cow-related accidents occur inside a building. When frightened, cows cause many crushing and trampling injuries. Kicking, butting, and hooking are other ways in which a cow may cause injury. Even the most gentle cow may become dangerous when she is trying to protect a calf. Special precautions should be used when working around a mother and her calf.

Some heifers and high-strung cows, especially those with sore udders, are easily irritated. Special attention should be given to housekeeping that can prevent accidents to cows involving their feet and udders. Loose boards should be removed; wires and glass cleared away. The control of flies is another way to cut down on irritation to cows. An irritated cow can be dangerous.

bulls

Most injuries from bulls are caused by goring, butting, hooking, and trampling. All bulls, even pets, can become dangerous and kill. They can be handled safely, however, in well-constructed pens. When possible they should be isolated in their own area with adequate shelter, feed, water, exercise, and breeding facilities.

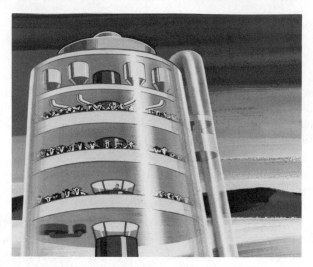

Figure 7-6. A high-rise feeder barn projected for the year 2000. Courtesy of Ford Motor Company, Tractor Operations.

feeder hogs

Most injuries with feeder hogs are caused by falling and trampling. Feeder hogs may attack people who are injured from some other source, especially if the person is bleeding.

sows

Sows are sometimes very cross and irritable around farrowing time and while their pigs are young.

herd sires

Herd sires should always receive special consideration. Whether stallion, ram, bull, or boar, they are capable of becoming very dangerous when in the presence of other sires of the same species. One should, for example, be very careful about putting two stallions in the same pen.

horses

Horses are easily startled by sudden noises. When that happens they may kick before looking. Kicking is a horse's best defense against danger. A good safety rule to remember is to always speak to a horse in a gentle manner when approaching it for any reason. Always speak to a horse, for example, before patting him on the rump. Safety-minded people never approach a horse from the rear if it is possible to do otherwise.

Horseback riding is a popular activity in this country. Safe riding habits are essential. Even the most experienced riders can suffer bad accidents when they become over-confident or inattentive. Horses respect firmness and seem to sense when an inexperienced rider is aboard. One should never ride a horse that is too spirited to handle; good riders, however, can and do ride spirited horses with safety. Inexperienced riders can suffer terrible tragedies from the most gentle horses.

Never mount a horse in a barn. Be sure all gear, such as stirrup leathers, bridles, reins, and cinches, is in good condition. They should be replaced when signs of wear become apparent. Riders should be alert at all times to the possibility of the horse's stumbling or being scared by a dog, snake, car, or some other source.

Probably the best advice that can be given is not to "over horse" yourself. Be sure you can handle the mount safely. If you are unsure, you should either not ride or seek the advice of an experienced person. Even this advice, unfortunately, can turn out wrong.[20]

animal diseases and man

Animals are a more common source of disease to humans than most people think. Of the slightly more than 200 diseases that affect human beings, more than 90 are transmitted by animals.[21] Farmers as a group have high exposure to various animals, so this fact alone makes animal-transmitted diseases a matter of serious concern to those interested in farm safety. Since many of the human diseases contracted from animals cannot be completely cured, prevention is of prime importance.[22]

Some examples of animal-related diseases capable of being transmitted to man are:

1. Brucellosis (Undulant or Malta fever in man), which affects the genital organs and causes sterility in both men and women.
2. Anthrax, which may enter the bloodstream and prove fatal.
3. Tularemia, causing chills, fever, and vomiting.
4. Newcastle disease, an infection transmitted from fowl.

[20] National Safety Council, *Safe Livestock Handling*, pamphlet (Chicago, n.d.), p. 4.

[21] National Safety Council, *Animal Disease and the Farmer*, pamphlet (Chicago, n.d.), p. 1.

[22] National Safety Council, *Animal Disease and the Farmer*, p. 1.

5. Trichinosis, an infestation of roundworms.
6. Rabies.
7. Bovine tuberculosis.

The incidence of two of these diseases—brucellosis and rabies—is very high. Brucellosis, for example, affects about 3.5 percent of all the cattle in the country and from 1 to 3 percent of all swine. It is most frequently transmitted to man by drinking raw milk from infected animals. As far as is known, brucellosis is not passed from person to person.[23]

Rabies is the most serious of all diseases transmitted by animal to man. The rabies virus enters the human body through a break in the skin, usually from a bite. There are thousands of rabies cases reported yearly among the animal population. The grim fact that makes rabies so serious in man is that unless serum is administered after a bite and before the disease begins, it is almost 100 percent fatal. Not long ago a patient in Ohio did survive a case of rabies, due to the efforts and alertness of a medical team that anticipated and treated the symptoms as they occurred.[24] However, usually the disease progresses through three stages—premonitory, excitation, and paralysis. In the premonitory phase, humans display restlessness, depression, and fear. Feverishness, respiratory difficulties, headaches, and nervous excitability characterize the second stage. Muscle spasms in the throat and other body parts resulting in convulsions, unconsciousness, and then death are the typical effects of the last stage.[25]

For prevention, people should know the symptoms of rabies as they appear in animals. Abnormal behavior or a sudden change in disposition are always reasons for suspicion, such as a normally quiet dog who becomes nervous and erratic. Animals that normally prowl at night, such as skunks and foxes, should be suspected if seen in the daytime.[26]

Animal-related diseases can have serious effects on the farming industry. People in farm work should thoroughly familiarize themselves with these hazards and understand the importance of prevention and treatment. Figure 7-7 shows the phases of prevention.

Personal protection by the farmer begins with adequate knowledge concerning disease prevention. It means proper sanitation, personal cleanliness, and other preventive measures, such as wearing protective gloves when handling the remains of suspect animals. It also means not drinking unpasteurized milk.

[23] National Safety Council, *Animal Disease and the Farmer,* p. 1.
[24] C. D. VanderMey, "Rabies Gone Wild," *Farm Safety Review,* September-October 1972, p. 12.
[25] VanderMey, "Rabies Gone Wild," p. 12.
[26] VanderMey, "Rabies Gone Wild," p. 13.

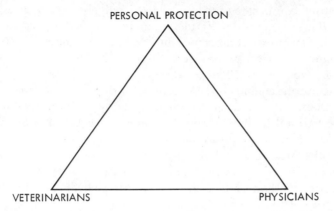

PERSONAL PROTECTION

VETERINARIANS   PHYSICIANS

Figure 7-7. Prevention triangle for animal-transmitted diseases. Adapted from the National Safety Council bulletin, Animal Disease and the Farmer.

The veterinarian can play an important role through proper diagnosis and recognition of these diseases. Inoculation, quarantine, and other procedures are good preventive methods.

The physician should be aware of animal-related diseases. He has various prevention and treatment procedures available. But in the final analysis the farmer must bear the main responsibility for his own safety, although he should seek the help and guidance of professionals. Proper prevention procedures can reduce the need for many countermeasures.

AGRICULTURAL CHEMICALS

Agricultural chemicals have many uses—to protect food, fiber, and other products from destruction by fungi, bacteria, viruses, insects, or rodents; as regulators of plant growth; and as plant nutrients or fertilizers. They are also used to protect the health of livestock and other animals.[27]

State and federal legislation, such as the Federal Environmental Pesticide Control Act of 1972, through the years has exercised control over these chemicals. Pesticides are a special type of agricultural chemical used to control insects, rodents, nematodes (worms), or other harmful pests. They are also used to eliminate undesired vegetation and to prevent or control the infection of plants by disease organisms such as viruses, fungi, and bacteria.[28] The pesticide act classified pesticides into two groups, those for restricted use and those for general use. Pesticides

[27] Manufacturing Chemists Association, Inc., *Agricultural Chemicals* (Washington, D. C., 1963), p. 35.
[28] Manufacturing Chemists Assn., *Agricultural Chemicals*, pp. 35–36.

in the restricted use category can be used only by certified applicators or under their supervision. Farmers can be certified to use them providing they can prove competence in handling the materials. Less hazardous materials that can be used safely with normal precautions are classified for general use.[29]

Agricultural chemicals represent a variety of potential hazards. Some are harmful only after entering the body in some manner, while others are harmful if they come into contact with the skin or eyes. The secret of safe handling and use of chemicals is in reading the labels and following the instructions carefully. Federal law requires that these chemicals be labeled with instructions for their safe use and storage.

The safe method of handling agricultural chemicals is determined by the nature of the chemical itself and is related to its method of causing harm. If necessary, special protective clothing should be worn. Figure 7-8 shows the proper clothing to be worn while working with highly toxic agricultural chemicals.

OTHER HAZARDS IN FARMING

Noise has been called the "third pollutant," following air and water pollution. Constant exposure to excessive noise can cause hearing loss. This is very common to farmers since they are overly exposed to noise while operating tractors and other heavy equipment. One recent study showed that farmers as a group have a greater loss of hearing than does the general public. They also suffer hearing losses in relation to the amount of time spent on a tractor.[30] Proper protective measures, such as ear muffs or plugs, can reduce hearing loss. Farm equipment manufacturers should make a concerted effort to reduce noise hazards.

Grain bins are another example of a hazard unique to the farmer. They are especially dangerous during unloading operations. Some grains such as flax are dangerous even when not unloading. A 12-year-old boy in Iowa climbed undetected into a grain bin during an emptying operation. The grain stopped flowing from the outlet, the first indication of trouble. A probe at the outlet chute exposed the boy's feet and legs. He had already suffocated by the time he was removed from the bin.[31]

Manure pits are a special problem. Four gases—ammonia, methane,

[29] National Safety Council, "Read the Label," *Farm Safety Review*, January-February 1973, p. 3.

[30] William J. Fletcher, "Noise—The Third Pollution," *Farm Safety Review*, March-April 1970, p. 11.

[31] W. D. Hanford, "Grain Bins Can Be Dangerous," *Farm Safety Review*, May-June 1970, p. 3.

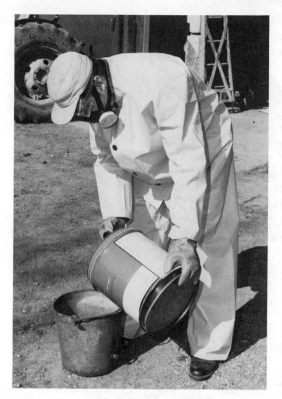

Figure 7-8. Protective clothing used in handling agricultural chemicals. Courtesy of the National Safety Council.

carbon dioxide, and hydrogen sulfide—are prevalent in manure regardless of the source. Only hydrogen sulfide is poisonous, but the others create serious problems. Many other organic gases are found in manure, but they seem to be offensive only because of their distinctive odor. People who work around manure storage tanks should exercise such precautions as never working alone, using lifelines, ventilating the tanks before entering, and testing for oxygen levels.[32]

Overexposure to the sun is always serious, regardless of the circumstances. The fact that a huge proportion of farm work is carried on outside during the summer months increases the danger of this hazard. Cancer of the skin increases dramatically among people who are consistently exposed to the sun. Farmers should take every precaution possible to keep their skin shaded as much as possible.

[32] William J. Fletcher, "Work Safely Around Manure Pits and Other Underground Tanks," *Farm Safety Review*, July-August 1969, p. 3.

Such highly flammable material as gasoline is often stored in an unsafe manner on farms. Figure 7-9 shows examples of safe and unsafe gasoline storage.

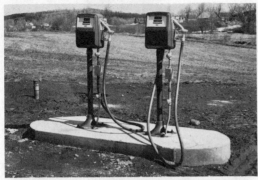

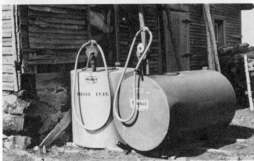

Figure 7-9. *(a) Safe and (b) unsafe gasoline storage. Courtesy of the National Safety Council.*

Exposure to dusts, chemicals which may be both toxic and irritating to the skin, and poisonous plants make the use of protective equipment a necessity on the farm. Figure 7-10 shows some examples of protective equipment in use on today's farms.

SUMMARY

Farm work accident rates rank third after mining and construction. Because of the number of skills he must have, the complexity of the tasks he must perform, and the highly sophisticated and diverse equipment he uses, a farmer has a hazardous occupation.

More adequate accident data and analysis are clearly needed to provide a basis for accident prevention programs. There have been recent gains in this area. We can reasonably expect the collection of accident data to become systemized on a national scale very soon.

4-H Clubs, other farm organizations, the manufacturers of farm

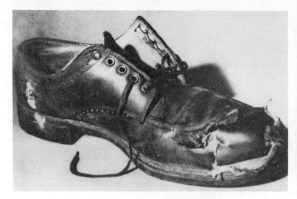

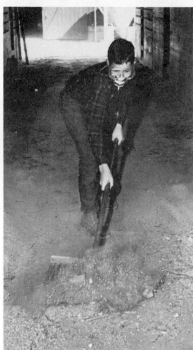

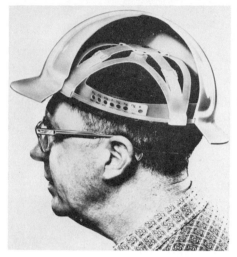

Figure 7-10. *Safety equipment used in farm operations. Courtesy of the National Safety Council.*

equipment, and interested agencies should step up their education and training programs, especially in the area of safe tractor operation.

Advanced technology, especially as it relates to human factors, should improve the safety features on farm equipment. The combination of all these things, if properly executed, should make possible reductions in farm accidents.

SUGGESTED STUDENT ACTIVITIES

1. Visit a farm and observe the highly sophisticated equipment in operation, and then make a list of the safety hazards you observed.
2. Do a task analysis of a farm procedure.
3. Have a representative from a 4-H Club or a county agent speak before your class.

4. Visit a meat-packing plant and see the safety precautions taken in the handling of meat.

5. If possible analyze an actual farm accident to determine proximate and contributing causes.

6. Write a paper on some phase of farm safety.

7. Make a film or slide-tape series showing modern farm equipment and explaining the safety hazards connected with the equipment, with suggested safeguards.

8. Visit a stockyard or farm and notice how the feed lots and pens are arranged for safety.

9. Design a well-laid-out feed lot and barn yard.

BIBLIOGRAPHY

Doss, Howard J., and Pfister, Richard G. *Nature and Extent of Farm Machinery Use in Relation to Frequency of Accidents.* Agricultural Engineering Department, Center for Rural Manpower and Public Affairs, Report No. 30. East Lansing, Michigan: Michigan State University, 1971, pp. 1, 6.

Fletcher, William J. "Avoiding Elevator and Auger Accidents." *Farm Safety Review,* November-December 1969, pp. 5–6.

———. "Noise—The Third Pollution." *Farm Safety Review,* March-April 1970, p. 11.

———. "Work Safely Around Manure Pits and Other Underground Tanks." *Farm Safety Review,* July-August 1969, p. 3.

Hanford, W. D. "Grain Bins Can Be Dangerous." *Farm Safety Review,* May-June 1970, p. 3.

Manufacturing Chemists Association, Inc. *Agricultural Chemicals.* Washington, D. C., 1963.

National Safety Council. *Accident Facts 1973 Edition.* Chicago, 1973.

———. *Animal Disease and the Farmer.* Pamphlet. Chicago, n.d.

———. *Farm and Ranch Safety Guide.* Chicago, 1973.

———. "Read the Label." *Farm Safety Review,* January-February 1973, p. 3.

———. *Safe Livestock Handling.* Pamphlet. Chicago, n.d.

———. *Safe Tractor Operation.* Rural Accident Prevention Bulletin. Chicago, n.d.

———. "Ten State Accident Survey." *Farm Safety Review,* May-June 1973, p. 9.

VanderMey, C. D. "Rabies Gone Wild." *Farm Safety Review,* September-October 1972, pp. 12–13.

8

recreational safety

More leisure time and recreational sites, better transportation facilities, and a higher standard of living are some of the things responsible for the tremendous growth of the recreation industry. This trend should continue as shorter work weeks, higher pay, and increased vacation times become more commonplace.

Admittedly, recreational pursuits have many advantages for people and are important to their well-being. However, safety should be a first consideration both in choosing and pursuing an activity. As more people participate in more activities and as more recreational sites become available, there will undoubtedly be an increase in accidental deaths and injuries resulting from recreation. Education offers the greatest opportunity for preventing accidents and making these activities more enjoyable.

Although any activity carries certain risks, with few exceptions the risks can be minimized by taking some simple precautions. People should participate only in activities that are within their own physical and emotional capabilities.

SMALL CRAFT SAFETY

In 1971 almost 9 million boats were in use in the United States, that number is increased by thousands every year. In a recent year 1,418 deaths resulted from boating accidents, according to the United States Coast

Guard. Included in this total were 1,305 drownings and 113 deaths from other causes. Of the 1,305 reported drownings, 270 victims did not have life-saving devices. Of those who did, 486 failed to use them. In the same year 4,762 boating accidents were reported, half in open motorboats. In over 50 percent of these accidents, the principal cause was operator error.[1]

The more common boat hazards include overloading, improper loading, improper movement, improper trip planning, and horseplay.[2] All of these hazards are the direct result of human error and unsafe acts.

A huge variety of boats come in various shapes and sizes today, many with unstable characteristics. People should seek expert advice from reliable dealers before purchasing or renting boats. The intended use of the boat is important, but there are many other considerations when purchasing a boat. Safety should be first. Special consideration should be given to the floating characteristics of a small craft. What happens when it capsizes or fills with water? Small craft should have sufficient buoyancy or flotation ability to remain in a horizontal upright position and support the weight of the motor, if any, and the crew. Preferably, buoyancy compartments should be filled with expanded foam.[3]

Weather is one of the big hazards in boating. Small craft, because they are less stable, are especially vulnerable to high waves in bad weather conditions. The United States Weather Bureau issues advisories and long-range forecasts. One should never use a boat when adverse weather is forecast, even if he feels that the boat is stable under such conditions. Many weather hazards could be eliminated through proper trip planning procedures.

Some additional tips for safe boating are:

1. Have life preservers aboard in sufficient quantity and quality (Coast Guard approved).
2. Check the boat for leaks and other defects before leaving shore. Remove any water in the boat, thus eliminating slipping hazards.
3. Rowboats should have strong oars in neat-fitting and securely attached oarlocks.
4. Small boats should have an extra oar or paddle and a bailing can.

---

[1] National Safety Council, *Small Craft,* Safety Education Data Sheet No. 28 (Chicago, n.d.).

[2] National Safety Council, *Small Craft.*

[3] Charles W. Russell, "Small Craft Safety," in *Sports Safety,* ed. C. P. Yost (Washington, D. C.: American Association for Health, Physical Education and Recreation, 1971), p. 194.

5. Be sure the transom is solid and sufficiently strong to secure the motor.
6. Have boat and motor thoroughly checked at the beginning of the season.
7. Motor driven craft should have fire extinguishers and tools to make minor adjustments aboard.
8. Reduce speed when passing bathing beaches, canoes, and other boats. Allow at least 100 feet from scuba diver flags. (This is a red flag with a white diagonal stripe from the upper left corner to the lower right corner.)
9. Practice with your boat in shallow water near shore.
10. Be sure you know how to handle the boat in rough water.
11. If someone falls overboard grab him quickly and hang on. Get him into a life preserver, if available, before trying to get him back in the boat.[4]

An awareness of boating regulations, proper procedures, and common sense cannot be overemphasized. Use the boat within your own limitations and within those of the boat itself. Study the boating manual carefully and gain your experience in a safe manner.

FISHING

The United States Census Bureau has identified some 28 million people as serious fishermen and another 45 million who fish on a casual basis every year.[5] Fishing is enjoyed by many groups, from the very young to the very old. Adding to its popularity is the fact that one can engage in fishing in many different ways—bank fishing, stream wading, boat fishing, ice fishing, night fishing, and deep sea fishing.

Fishing would appear to be safer than other water sports, such as swimming or water skiing, yet it accounts for approximately 55 percent of the fatal boating accidents, whereas water skiing accounts for less than 5 percent. Boating accidents account for most fatal accidents in fishing, but hooks and poles, in that order, are responsible for most injuries. Certain fish such as catfish and bullheads have dangerous pectoral and dorsal fins, while large game fish such as muskellunge and pike have very sharp teeth. A combination of factors—boats, the water, equipment dangers,

[4] National Safety Council, *Small Craft.*
[5] National Safety Council, "Fishing—Biggest Boating Danger," *Family Safety Magazine,* Spring 1967, p. 4.

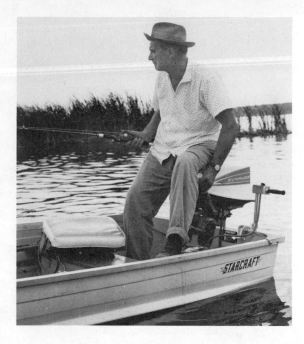

Figure 8-1. *A trademark of the professional fishing guide: sitting on the motor. Don't try to imitate him. You're not the old pro he is, and you can prove your amateur status quickly if you hit a rock or snag. Photo courtesy of the National Safety Council.*

fish hazards, and the unsafe acts of fishermen—combine to provide a high-risk situation in many cases.[6]

Not only does fishing provide excellent recreational benefits, but it also has the added incentive of a tasty meal if the catch is good. The sport is quite safe if proper precautions such as the following are taken:

1. Be careful when casting, especially when in a boat with others or in crowded quarters. Overhead casting is the most accurate and the safest method.
2. Remain seated in a boat or be sure someone else remains seated to steady the boat if you have to change positions.
3. If you wish to change positions with someone, return to shore or shallow water.
4. Load the boat carefully with proper equipment such as life preservers.
5. Be on the lookout for storms. Head for shore immediately in case of a storm threat.
6. Be sure the boat and motor match.
7. Never sit on a motor when fishing.
8. Be sure you have an ample gas supply and lights for running after dark.
9. Know how to bait hooks properly and how to remove fish from the hooks.

[6] National Safety Council, *Fishing*, Safety Education Data Sheet No. 44 (Chicago, n.d.).

10. If ice fishing, check with local authorities about ice conditions. Watch for carbon monoxide in tents.
11. Never wade in a stream when alone and watch for slippery rocks and underwater snags and hazards.[7]

The risk of boating accidents must be minimized. Be sure you have a thorough knowledge of boat operations, including boating regulations, before leaving shore. Fishing can be fun and exciting—and very safe, if common sense is used.

WATER SKIING

The thrill of water skiing attracts several million participants who purchase hundreds of thousands of water skis each year. The sport is safe and healthful. Skiers do get their share of dramatic dunkings, but this is not dangerous if a person knows what he is doing.[8] Apparently the most dangerous act is operating the towing boat. It is there, according to recent Coast Guard figures, that more than 17 percent of all boating injuries (not deaths) occur. That is a high injury rate when one considers exposure, since there are millions of boats used for purposes other than

[7] National Safety Council, *Fishing.*
[8] Laura O'Connell, "Danger Rides in the Boat," *Family Safety Magazine,* Spring 1966, p. 4.

Figure 8-2. Avoid precarious reaching and balancing to get unhooked after a bad cast. A sudden movement, a hard turn, accidentally throwing the motor in reverse, hitting a rock or snag—all make standing risky at any time. Photo courtesy of the National Safety Council.

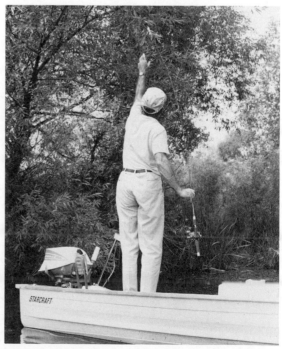

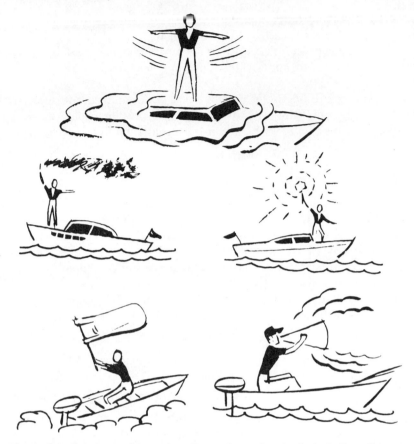

Figure 8-3. Boating safety: when in trouble—signal, don't holler. Courtesy of the National Safety Council.

skiing.[9] Towing skiers is not an easy task and requires alertness, skill, perception, and knowledge of boating regulations. The operator of the boat must not only watch the skier, but must also be on the lookout for other boats.[10] Water skiing does require the use of safety precautions.

Some additional recommended safety actions are:

1. Be a good swimmer.
2. Wear a flotation device, preferably a life jacket, even if you are an experienced swimmer.
3. Have either a wide angle mirror on the boat or an experienced observer aboard.

[9] O'Connell, "Danger Rides in the Boat," p. 4.
[10] O'Connell, "Danger Rides in the Boat," p. 4.

4. Stop the motor when the skier is entering the boat.
5. Avoid piers, floats, other boats, fishermen, swimming beaches, buoyed channels, and boat anchorages.
6. Watch the water ahead.
7. Obtain proper equipment and check it often.
8. Follow standard procedures and know the meaning of hand signals.
9. Avoid skiing after dark.[11]

Several states have enacted codes regarding water skiing. Skiers and boat operators should be familiar with their state codes.

SWIMMING

Swimming has always been a, if not *the*, most popular form of outdoor recreation. Increases in swimming facilities, longer vacations, and better transportation keep it popular.[12] It is both a competitive and a recreational activity with lifetime benefits, and it is generally recognized as one of the best all-around types of exercise.

If current projections hold true, swimming will continue to increase in popularity. There is thus a need for stepped-up educational programs teaching people to swim and developing proper attitudes and understandings concerning the potential dangers. This must begin with home effort, with the parents being sure that adequate instruction is provided. The ease and safety with which young children can be taught to swim makes this early teaching desirable.

In 1969, 7,300 persons drowned; about 2,800 deaths resulted from swimming or playing in the water. The remaining 4,500 drownings were non-swimming fatalities—persons falling into the water from bridges or docks, and so forth.[13] Probably many of the 4,500 deaths could have been prevented if the people had been able to swim with some degree of proficiency. In 1972, 7,600 lives were lost through drowning accidents, making drowning the third largest cause of accidental death after motor vehicle accidents and falls.[14]

There are many agencies, such as schools, the YMCA, and YWCA, the American Red Cross, and others, that offer swimming instructions. Most progressive park recreational programs also provide swimming lessons.

[11] O'Connell, "Danger Rides in the Boat," p. 5.
[12] National Safety Council, *Swimming*, Safety Education Data Sheet No. 27 (Chicago, n.d.).
[13] National Safety Council, *Swimming*.
[14] National Safety Council, *Accident Facts 1973 Edition* (Chicago, 1973), p. 6.

The large number of swimming places makes education the key to preventing deaths by drowning. There are literally millions of unguarded swimming areas along our nation's streams, as well as in ponds and small lakes, and the number has increased in recent years due to conservation efforts. All of these unimproved areas represent exceptional dangers. Add the public beaches, public swimming pools, motel pools, and the increasing number of home pools, and the result is a very complex network of swimming facilities.

Home pools have been dropped by the thousands into a society that is not trained or equipped to deal with their possible dangers. There is really no effective way to place controls on all of the potential danger spots; thus education is the only possible way to create the most meaningful safety efforts in swimming.

Many other factors in swimming make the sport hazardous, such as the swimmer's inability to withstand the effects of cold temperatures, or swimming without proper equipment, as so often happens in salt water where distance swimmers require goggles. The tendency to overestimate one's ability or physical stamina is also a major contributing factor in swimming accidents.

People should either learn minimum swimming skills or avoid water hazards. With adequate instruction and proper consideration for one's ability and physical limitations, the sport is perfectly safe. Without question the potential benefits from swimming, when the risk is minimized, outweigh the potential dangers.

Some safe swimming tips are:

1. Physical exams are a good idea, especially for older and more sedentary individuals.
2. Swim only in protected areas and obey the rules.
3. Know and observe your own swimming capabilities and limitations.
4. Use the buddy system. Never swim alone.
5. Keep away from swift moving water and be alert for undertow. If caught in current swim with it and at the same time angle toward shore.
6. Do not dive, wade, or swim into places of unknown depths or where there may be hidden rocks, sudden drop-offs, or strong currents.
7. Keep hands off others in deep water. Before venturing into deep water know how to swim, tread water, and execute turns.
8. Stay out of water during thunderstorms. Keep calm if you are having difficulty.[15]

[15] National Safety Council, *Swimming.*

CAMPING

According to the Bureau of Outdoor Recreation, by 1980 camping activity will show a 78 percent increase over 1965.[16] The growing popularity of this leisure-time activity is due to many factors, such as the accessibility of camp sights, good camping equipment produced on a mass basis, and the increased amount of leisure time.

Today's camper is no longer dependent on a tent or cabin for shelter. He has at his disposal, on a purchase or rental basis, a variety of motorized equipment ranging from small trailers and campers mounted on small trucks to larger, more sophisticated travel homes. The camper can bring many of the conveniences of the modern home to the campground.

Today's camper can take his choice from youth camps, day camps, those designed for the entire family, camps operated by youth groups, church groups, schools, colleges, and private organizations. Many camps offer planned and well-organized recreational programs. Boating, fishing, scuba diving, hiking, golf, tennis, horseback riding, and many other activities are common.

Since camping does not fall into a nationally organized category for accident classification, there are no national accident statistics available. Fatalities occurring in camping activities are categorized as drownings, falls, and boating accidents, and therefore are not charged directly to camping activities.[17]

Good pre-trip planning is an essential element in making the camping excursion safe and enjoyable. There are many guidebooks and pamphlets available to aid the prospective camper in the planning process. The type of camp selected will determine the kinds of equipment and clothing needed. All equipment should be checked before leaving. Some authorities suggest a trial run in the backyard.

The hazards of camping include such things as poisonous plants, insects and reptiles, wild animals, fire and exposure. Getting lost is a common occurrence. All campers should be equipped with compasses, if possible, and a knowledge of how to handle themselves when lost.

For unorganized camping groups, the American Camping Association recommends that one adult accompany every four children. It also recommends a maximum of eight campers under one adult's supervision.[18]

Without question, camping will continue to increase in popularity.

[16] National Safety Council, Camping, Safety Education Data Sheet No. 18 (Chicago, n.d.).

[17] National Safety Council, Camping.

[18] National Safety Council, Camping.

The more people participating, the more accidental deaths and injuries. Safety is a prerequisite to enjoyable camping. Some additional hints to encourage safe camping are:

1. Do not swim in unsupervised areas.
2. Camp only in designated areas.
3. Never feed wild animals.
4. Maintain first aid equipment in top-notch condition.
5. Supervise young children carefully.
6. Use fires for a purpose, such as cooking or heating, and use prescribed methods of control.[19]

.   *HUNTING*

Hunting is one of the oldest sports known to man. Early man had to hunt for survival; in many cases it provided his main source of food. The tradition remains, and today millions of people engage in hunting for recreation and food (the tasty wildlife dish).

Most hunting accidents originate from two sources—firing a gun on purpose and firing a gun accidentally. Those caused by firing a gun intentionally occur in several different ways: shooting someone when firing at a moving target; firing in the direction of sound without identifying the source; bullets richocheting; bullets going beyond their intended target; failing to check if a gun is loaded; using the wrong ammunition; and using a faulty gun.[20] A gun can be accidentally fired by dropping or bumping it, or by catching the trigger on some object.[21] Hunting therefore requires extreme care and concern for others.

Although firearms are discussed in the chapter on home safety, these are some additional hints for hunting safety:

1. When selecting a hunting partner use the same criteria you would use in rating yourself on hunting safety.
2. Wear the proper color of clothing as prescribed by local authorities.
3. Be absolutely sure of your target before you pull the trigger. Know the identifying features of your target.

[19] Herbert J. Stack and J. Duke Elkow, *Education for Safe Living*, 4th ed. (Englewood Cliffs, N. J.: Prentice-Hall, Inc., © 1966), p. 94.
[20] Louis F. Lucas, "Hunting and Shooting," in *Sports Safety*, ed. C. P. Yost (Washington, D. C.: American Association for Health, Physical Education and Recreation, 1971), p. 255.
[21] Lucas, "Hunting and Shooting," p. 255.

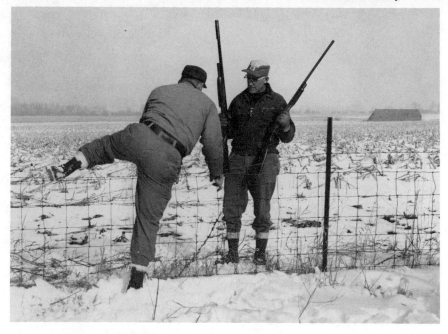

Figure 8-4. *These hunters are taking proper safety precautions for crossing a fence. Photo courtesy of the National Safety Council.*

4. Never climb a tree or fence or jump a ditch with a loaded gun.
5. Drink no alcoholic beverages before or during the hunting session.[22]

SNOWMOBILES

Snowmobiles are actually motor vehicles. They have a low horsepower engine and are designed primarily for travel on snow or ice.[23] The engine power is transferred into an endless track made of a rubber-like flexible material with many cleats of steel. Depending on design, these little machines are capable of developing high speeds. The running speed can be as low as 4 or 5 miles per hour, and cruising speed in light snow ranges from 20 to 30 mph, but snowmobiles have been clocked at speeds of 65 mph.[24]

[22] National Safety Council, *Firearms*, Safety Education Data Sheet No. 3 (Chicago, n.d.).
[23] National Safety Council, *Snowmobiles*, Safety Education Data Sheet No. 100 rev. (Chicago, n.d.).
[24] National Safety Council, "Meet the Snowmobile," *Family Safety Magazine*, Winter 1967, p. 13.

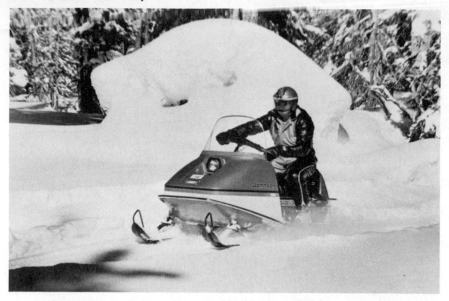

Figure 8-5. *A snowmobile in operation. Photo courtesy of Johnson Snowmobile Division.*

In the 1971-72 season snowmobile accidents killed 164 people. Collisions with fixed objects accounted for 52 deaths. Unsuitable terrain contributed to 13 deaths. In these cases the victims drove off cliffs, were thrown from their vehicle, or were crushed by the snowmobile. Ice breakthroughs resulted in 21 deaths.[25]

Due to the increasing numbers of snowmobiles, many states have enacted legislation concerning their operation. Operators must be aware of these regulations. Snowmobiles are valuable pieces of equipment and have many uses. They are especially valuable for rescue work, since they can travel to out-of-the-way places under difficult circumstances. They are a functional piece of equipment in many northern states. Their recreational value includes joy riding, tobogganing, and pulling skiers.

The minimum safety equipment on a snowmobile includes properly functioning brake and steering systems, front and rear lights, and a rear view mirror. Brakes should always be checked at low speeds to be sure they are working correctly.[26]

Many safety rules concern snowmobile use. Operators would be well advised to read their operator manuals carefully and practice with the machines at low speeds, learning the capabilities of turning, stopping,

[25] National Safety Council, *Snowmobiles.*
[26] National Safety Council, *Snowmobiles.*

and so on. One should gain his experience with these machines slowly and carefully.

GOLF

Once only a rich man's game, golf is now popular with men and women from all levels of society. It is common practice, especially in highly populated areas, to require tee-time reservations at courses, especially on weekends. The number of golf courses has increased in the last few years, but they have still failed to keep up with the demand. Better transportation and television coverage of golfing events have helped to promote the sport's popularity. It can be played by young and old, and has health and recreational benefits.

There are no accurate statistics covering the number of injuries or deaths sustained through golf, but scores of people are injured annually, some of them fatally.

Golf is a game that requires good physical conditioning for safe participation. Few people appreciate the fine conditioning necessary for the players on the pro tour. Heart attack and heat exhaustion caused by overexertion are common to golfers. Golfing enthusiasts should condition themselves before attempting long, hard rounds of golf. An adequate warm-up is essential, especially for the occasional golfer.

Common courtesy will prevent many golf injuries. Waiting until golfers in front of you are well out of range before hitting is an example. Survey the situation before you hit, and determine whether other people are within range of your shot, allowing for hooks and slices. The rule that the person farthest from the pin hits first is a common sense safety rule, as well as a courtesy.

Only take practice swings in designated areas or when it is your time to hit, and then check to see if someone is close to you. Always stand behind the person who is hitting.

The golf ball coming from nowhere is a source of many injuries. A well-hit drive may travel upward of 250 mph. Fortunately most golf balls lose much of their velocity before they hit someone. One of the factors in choosing a course to play should be the physical layout. Some courses have narrow fairways with no tree protection in between, with players hitting in close quarters. Physical layout can make a golf course dangerous.

Golf carts are a source of many injuries. The American Golf Cart Manufacturers Association is in the process of developing standards for golf carts. Some carts have poor stability, poor braking systems, or poor steering mechanisms. Insufficient maintenance is oftentimes a factor in golf cart instability. Extreme care should be used crossing narrow bridges or traveling on the sides of hills. Golf carts should be operated at safe speeds and with common sense.

Weather can be a hazard on a golf course, especially during lightning. Never seek shelter under a lone tree. Golf carts and golf equipment should be avoided during electrical storms. Seek shelter in a ravine or building if possible. A golfer standing alone on a fairway is an easy target for lightning.

PRIVATE FLYING

There is considerable disagreement in the statistics concerning private flying, but all indicate that it is much safer than many people believe. General aviation in the United States has grown tremendously in the last few years. The aircraft industry has responded to user demand and has produced a variety of aircraft suitable for different purposes.

Stringent regulations govern flying, including rigid physical examinations for crew members. The regulations cover all phases of aircraft operation. The government in turn provides many excellent services to pilots, mainly in the form of weather forecasts and advisories and air-traffic control.

Today's private pilots are flying aircraft with higher speeds than some World War II aircraft. They do so safely under the watchful eye of the Federal Aviation Administration, which governs flight standards. Today's private pilot is better trained than those in past years. By law, the private pilot must now have a sound understanding of the principles of flight, weather, aircraft engine operation, flight instruments, radio communications, and flight planning. His aircraft in most cases is equipped with sophisticated navigation equipment, which is sensitive to a nation-wide network of aircraft navigation signals.

Most accidents are the result of pilot error, many occurring on the ground prior to takeoff. Most errors occur in improper flight planning, failure to check weather conditions, and gambling on weather conditions at the point of destination or along the way. Adequate pre-flight inspection of the aircraft will normally turn up any defects that need correction before flight. It is the pilot who fails to exercise precautions or fails to heed pre-flight warning indications who usually ends up in trouble.

Many simple precautions in flight will avoid accidents. For example, never fly a single-engine plane over large bodies of water even if equipped to do so; never fly directly over big cities in single-engine aircraft; and avoid flying single-engine aircraft at night. Maintain sufficient altitude so that you have plenty of time to execute a safe landing in case of engine failure. Single-engine airplanes are among the safest if operated properly. They have a gliding capacity that enables one to reach a safe landing spot in most cases, especially if sufficient altitude is maintained during normal flight.

Weather is the biggest hazard, so the pilot must understand and appreciate weather phenomena. Ability to navigate is imperative and will be enhanced by proper pre-flight planning. Good pilots are safe pilots. They do not endanger themselves or their passengers and enjoy the thrill and satisfaction of safe flying.

SUMMARY

Participation in recreational activities has grown tremendously in recent years. This growth should continue as society becomes more affluent, as people have increased leisure time, and as more recreational sites are developed. With increased participation we can expect increases in accidental deaths and injuries resulting from the activities, unless suitable countermeasures can be developed.

The increasing number of recreational sites and the thousands of possible swimming places preclude the development of supervisory methods and personnel for adequate coverage. Therefore education must play the key role in minimizing the accident problem in recreation. Schools and other interested agencies will have to increase their efforts in this direction.

Recreation plays an important role in allowing man to escape from his daily routines. It plays an important role in the mental health of our nation as well as in preserving the family unit. We must make these activities as safe as possible. To do otherwise makes them self-defeating.

SUGGESTED STUDENT ACTIVITIES

1. Plan a recreational outing for a group of four people, including travel, routing and equipment needed. (Analyze all possible hazards and show countermeasures.)
2. Survey at least two recreational sites for possible hazards, and plan workable countermeasures.
3. Do a task analysis of a recreational activity.
4. As a class, develop the plans for a "safety clinic" in some recreational activity, such as swimming or fishing.
5. Invite a recreational expert to appear before your class and talk on safety.

BIBLIOGRAPHY

LUCAS, LOUIS F. "Hunting and Shooting." In *Sports Safety,* edited by C. P. Yost. Washington, D. C.: American Association for Health, Physical Education and Recreation, 1971.

NATIONAL SAFETY COUNCIL. *Accident Facts 1973 Edition.* Chicago, 1973.

————. *Camping.* Safety Education Data Sheet No. 18. Chicago, n.d.

————. *Firearms.* Safety Education Data Sheet No. 3. Chicago, n.d.

————. *Fishing.* Safety Education Data Sheet No. 44. Chicago, n.d.

————. "Fishing—Biggest Boating Danger." *Family Safety Magazine,* Spring 1967, p. 4.

————. "Meet the Snowmobile." *Family Safety Magazine,* Winter 1967, p. 13.

————. *Small Craft.* Safety Education Data Sheet No. 28. Chicago, n.d.

————. *Snowmobiles.* Safety Education Data Sheet No. 100 rev. Chicago, n.d.

————. *Swimming.* Safety Education Data Sheet No. 27. Chicago, n.d.

O'CONNELL, LAURA. "Danger Rides in the Boat." *Family Safety Magazine,* Spring 1968, p. 4.

RUSSELL, CHARLES W. "Small Craft Safety." In *Sports Safety,* edited by C. P. Yost. Washington, D. C.: American Association for Health, Physical Education and Recreation, 1971.

STACK, HERBERT J., and ELKOW, J. DUKE. *Education for Safe Living.* 4th ed. Englewood Cliffs, N. J.: Prentice-Hall, Inc., 1966.

9

school safety education

Safety and safety education are the responsibility of the individual board of education and school administration. They have a moral and legal responsibility to maintain a school environment that is as safe as possible from environmental hazards. At the same time they must offer students planned educational opportunities to develop optimal habits, skills, attitudes, and knowledge related to safe and effective living.

Poorly developed or non-existent safety programs exact a very high price in terms of loss of life, injury, and suffering. The public has the right and the responsibility to hold the board of education accountable for these failures. As in industrial safety programs, the key to success is communication, responsibility, and accountability.

Despite legislation in every state, safety education and safe school environments are often only secondary considerations. Admittedly the various elements in the total educational curriculum compete strenuously for the attention and support of school administrators. Nevertheless there should be balance in the curriculum.

For years safety and safety education have received less attention than they deserve. This neglect results in the needless loss of thousands of lives annually through accidents. Although we do not know how many of these lives could have been saved with proper education, every fact points to the conclusion that failure to develop proper habits, skills, attitudes, and knowledge is the real culprit. How long can we afford this loss, when a few minutes spent daily in the classroom in well-planned safety education programs could probably save so many?

Many educators' attitudes toward safety are evident in textbooks on curriculum or school construction. Some of these books do not even mention the word "safety" nor is it found in the subject indexes.

All too often safety functions are relegated to a committee within the school system. Committees are important. They can and do offer valuable advice and direction, especially toward curriculum construction. In most cases, however, they cannot effectively administer a safety program or a safety education program in a school system. That responsibility should be given to an individual who is trained in safety and safety education. Such experts should work with the various committees in the school system and with community agencies; but they must have the necessary authority to activate and develop programs consistent with educational policies in their particular system, and they must in turn be held accountable.

More definitive school policies toward safety and safety education, with assigned responsibility and accountability, will begin to diminish the safety neglect in American education.

COOPERATION WITH OUTSIDE AGENCIES

All segments of society have a stake in school safety. Many private, voluntary, and governmental agencies outside the school work in the general safety area. They include:

1. *Industrial*—commercial groups.
2. *Voluntary*—safety councils and professional organizations.
3. *Governmental*—police and fire departments, safety commissions, health departments, and others.[1]

In almost every community there are agencies and individuals who can make worthwhile contributions to accident prevention. Their interest can be nurtured and developed into a meaningful resource for the school system. The guidance and cooperation of these groups should be vigorously solicited by schools that desire a top grade safety program.

Cooperation between outside agencies and schools can be beneficial in several areas, including matters relating to:

[1] National Safety Council, "Work Together," *Safety Education*, September 1960, p. 10.

1. Safety education of the students.
2. Safe school environment, including to-and-from-school problems.
3. Public support for accident prevention.
4. Total community concern, for which the school, as an agency in the community, has a vital part.
5. Safe conduct of children throughout the community.[2]

SAFETY EDUCATION IN THE
SCHOOL CURRICULUM

Safety education has been defined in Chapter 1 as the sum of experiences which favorably affects the development of habits, skills, attitudes, and knowledge conducive to safe behavior. If the experience does not have a favorable effect, it becomes a deterrent to safety education. Children need experiences that will enable them to live and function safely in dangerous places. They must therefore develop judgment and self-guidance abilities.[3] Conservation of human resources and materials is the ultimate purpose of developing safe behavior in children. To achieve this in our modern, fast-moving society, curriculum development should be an ever-changing process, with provisions for reeducating people, as our technological advances cause them to change jobs and face new hazards.

Ross L. Neagley and N. Dean Evans succinctly described the necessity of maintaining a current and modern curriculum when they said:

> Each generation believes its problems are more difficult than those faced by previous generations. Too frequently, man looks backward for solutions to present day problems and while he searches in the past other new problems arise. The world moves on, time passes swiftly by, and the environment of today's children is vastly different from that of yesterday's. Tomorrow's children will feel the influences of even more fantastic changes.[4]

This constant change has special meaning for those in the field of curriculum development in safety education. Every new technological advance brings new hazards with which man must cope. This is a space-age society, and it is impossible to predict accurately the types of skills

---

[2] National Safety Council, "Work Together," p. 10.
[3] Laura Zirbes, "How Shall We Teach Them Safety?" *School Safety* 4, No. 2 (January-February 1969), p. 5.
[4] Ross L. Neagley and N. Dean Evans, *Handbook for Effective Curriculum Development* (Englewood Cliffs, N. J.: Prentice-Hall, Inc., © 1967), p. 35.

and knowledge that will be required in the future. Therefore a periodic reevaluation of curriculums should be routine procedure. Today's knowledge can no longer be used as the basis for curriculum.[5]

The American Association of School Administrators lists the following as "imperatives in education":

1. To strengthen the moral fabric of society.
2. To prepare people for the world of work.
3. To make intelligent use of our natural resources.
4. To discover and nurture creative talent.
5. To keep democracy working.
6. To deal constructively with psychological tensions.
7. To make the best use of leisure time.
8. To make urban life rewarding and satisfying.
9. To work with other people of the world for human betterment.[6]

This list makes obvious the fact that safety and safety education are "imperative" in a school program. Such education prepares people to recognize and meet the dangers of work. It deals with human betterment and makes life more rewarding. Safety education has proven its worth many times over. It is compatible with the school curriculum and always has been.

GUIDING PRINCIPLES FOR CURRICULUM CONSTRUCTION

Effective planning for safety education begins with a statement of policy by the board of education and school administration. The safety program should be planned in accordance with the curriculum pattern used for that particular school system. Safety education fits well into all types of curriculum patterns, whether child-centered, community-centered, or anything else. Most important—there must be some kind of planning for safety instruction.

The following principles are suggested for curriculum workers in safety education:

1. The safety education curriculum should be compatible with the total school curriculum.

[5] Neagley and Evans, *Handbook for Effective Curriculum Development*, p. 35.
[6] American Association of School Administrators, *Imperatives in Education* (Washington, D. C., 1966), p. i.

2. It must meet the needs of the learner.
3. The safety education curriculum must be designed to meet the needs of an ever-changing society.
4. It must be constantly evaluated and revised to meet the needs of the student and of society.
5. It should call for well-planned and desirable safety education experiences based on the best available knowledge at the time.
6. It must be allocated enough time.
7. Adequate budget provision must be made.
8. The safety education curriculum should be designed to provide for integration opportunities within other subjects.
9. It should be positive in nature.
10. The safety education curriculum should be designed to develop self-reliance in students.
11. The main goal is the development of safe behavior under all circumstances.
12. Psychologists and other specialists should evaluate the methods and materials to see that they are well suited to the age level of the children who will use them.

These principles are not exhaustive. Others pertinent to the particular school system should also be utilized.

Planning the safety education curriculum for the various grade levels should follow certain designated and logical steps. Phasing for curriculum development is illustrated in Figure 9-1.

STEP NO. 1	STEP NO. 2	STEP NO. 3	STEP NO. 4
DETERMINE	DEVELOP OBJECTIVES	RELATE	SELECT
THE NEEDS OF SOCIETY THE NEEDS OF THE LEARNER	SKILLS NEEDED HABITS NEEDED KNOWLEDGES NEEDED ATTITUDES NEEDED	INTEREST OF THE LEARNER ABILITIES OF THE LEARNER	LEARNING EXPERIENCES COURSE CONTENT BASED ON VALID AND UP-TO-DATE INFORMATION TEACHING METHODS

Figure 9-1. *Phasing of curriculum development.*

the safety education curriculum committee

The safety education curriculum committee should be made up of representatives from the various subject areas in the school. It should also include representatives from the administration, parent groups, students, and interested community agencies. Committee makeup will be influenced by the community and type of school for which the curriculum is designed. Figure 9-2 illustrates a suggested curriculum committee.

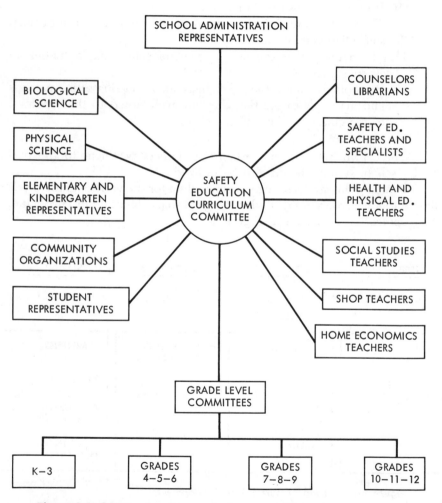

Figure 9-2. Safety education curriculum committee.

DETERMINING THE NEEDS OF
SOCIETY AND THE LEARNER

The needs of society and the learner are constantly changing. This fact, along with the current explosion of knowledge and technological advances, makes curriculum development, evaluation, and revision a continuous process. The safety needs of society and the learner can be determined by several different methods, such as:

1. Analysis of accidents.
2. Analysis of student activities.
3. Analysis of environmental hazards.[7]

analysis of accidents

Accidents in the home, community, and school should provide clues to what types of instruction are needed to develop the habits, skills, knowledge, and attitudes necessary to combat them. A study of the accident patterns may determine the timing of instruction. Many accidents are seasonal; instructional patterns should be geared to these variations as much as possible.

Adequate school and community accident reports are a necessity. The starting point for any good school safety program is the accident record-keeping system. It will tell you where you are and where you need to go. Accident record systems provide the basis for remedial programming.

analysis of student activities

As students grow and develop, their types of activities change. An analysis of student activities will show the types of possible hazards, and perhaps will provide hints for accident prevention.

analysis of environmental hazards

An analysis of environmental hazards can provide a basis for removing at least some of those hazards, and it can show ways of reducing the chances of accidents where the hazards are impossible to

---

[7] Herbert J. Stack and J. Duke Elkow, *Education for Safe Living*, 4th ed. (Englewood Cliffs, N. J.: Prentice-Hall, Inc., © 1966), p. 231.

remove. Remember, no environment can be made completely free of hazards. Instead, we must control the hazards and instill self-reliance and confidence in students, so that they can be successful in dealing with the hazards that do exist.

other methods of determining needs

Communitywide safety surveys and interviews with parents and community leaders will provide insights into the needs of the society in that particular community. The students themselves should be surveyed and their desires and opinions weighed by people in curriculum construction.

DEVELOPING OBJECTIVES OF THE
SAFETY EDUCATION PROGRAM

Once the needs of society and the learner are known, the curriculum planner can determine appropriate objectives. Some suggested principles for developing objectives are:

1. They should be specific in terms of habits, attitudes, skills, and knowledge as they relate to safe behavior.
2. They should be meaningful to the students, who should see personal benefits in gaining the stated objectives.
3. Objectives should be attainable by the learners for which they are intended. They should match skill capabilities.
4. They should be compatible with the overall objectives of the community's educational system.
5. They should be measurable to every extent possible, and they should be performance based.

The measurement and evaluation of objectives related to knowledge are fairly simple provided that the tests are relevant to the material used in the learning process. Statistical analysis can determine the validity and reliability of written testing devices.

The measurement of behavioral objectives is not as easy. Industry has been somewhat successful in evaluating on-the-spot responses to different situations. We must learn to make use of this type of technique if we are to assess the effectiveness of our teaching.[8] Parents and teachers

[8] Norman Key, "Safety Education," in *Curriculum Handbook for School Executives*, ed. William J. Ellena (Washington, D. C.: American Association of School Administrators, 1973), p. 283.

should observe the child. Specially prepared checklists would make attempts to measure behavioral goals more objective.

Attitudes are still more difficult to measure. They are, as we know, predispositions to act and to that degree can be subjectively observed and recorded. Attitudes are expressed in the behavior of the individual.

determining the interests of the student

Student interests may be determined in a variety of ways—through interest inventories, surveys, discussions with parents, and other methods. People tend to be interested in their own needs. Thus if we know the needs, then it follows that interest should be high, provided that instructional materials and methods are compatible with those needs. The good teacher discovers individual interests and capitalizes on them to develop safe behavior. Every person wants to avoid injury and at the same time enjoy activity. Maximum enjoyment comes with adjusting and modifying behavior.

abilities

Ability comes in two distinct forms—comprehension, or mental ability, and motor ability. The rate of mental and physical development will be determined by these two abilities, and all objectives in the curriculum should be correlated with them. The good teacher can provide physical and mental activities to meet the range of individual abilities in a given classroom. The really good teacher uses the child's individual interests to motivate him or her toward higher goals.

SELECTION OF COURSE CONTENT

Selecting course content should be an ongoing process. Yesterday's knowledge cannot be the sole basis for the content of today's courses. Today's knowledge will not fulfill the needs of tomorrow. Man is doubling his knowledge every few years.

Certain principles, however, can be used in the selection of content and materials. Some suggested principles are:

1. The material must be modern and up to date.
2. Historical material should be used as it relates to the understanding of today's knowledge.
3. It should be appropriate for the intended grade level.
4. It should challenge the student.

5. It should be factual and scientific.
6. It should relate to the needs, interests, and comprehension abilities of the child.

SELECTION OF TEACHING METHODS

The needs, interests, and comprehension abilities of the children should determine the selection of teaching methods. In the final analysis the teachers must make the selection. They must choose those methods which they can best use and use comfortably. The good teacher employs many different methods. Variation tends to motivate students and to reinforce learning. Too many teachers use a "shotgun" approach, covering a lot of material while using very few methods. The reverse should be the case. Teachers should teach less, but carefully selected, material, and use several different methods or approaches.

There is general confusion concerning teaching aids. A teaching aid is an instrument used with a particular method of presentation. For instance, a projector is not a teaching method, but an instrument used in the audio-visual method of presentation. Several different methods of presentation should be available to teachers so that they can select those they feel are most suitable for the material and the learner.

Some examples of teaching methods are the following:

1. Demonstration.
2. Problem solving.
3. Dramatization and role playing.
4. Lecture.
5. Discussion.
6. Programmed or individualized instruction.
7. Group activities and committees.
8. Field trips.
9. Guest speakers.
10. Individual projects.
11. Audio-visual.
12. Question and answer.
13. Panel discussions.
14. Practice exercises, learning by doing.

Much research has been done on the validity of various teaching methods. Basically the teaching should be child-centered, not teacher-centered, for maximum effectiveness. The students must be actively engaged in the learning process. Child-centered activities require much preplanning by the teacher. This is probably the reason that so many teachers tend to make their presentations teacher-centered.

The teaching methods most often abused are lecture and audio-visual. The lecture is an excellent teaching method, providing that it is short in duration and stimulating. It is especially good for introducing material. However, it is too often overused because of lack of creativity on the part of the teacher. Students are in a "passive" situation during lectures; they should be actively engaged in the learning process. (This method is practically useless at the lower grade levels.)

Audio-visual techniques are excellent, but too many teachers rely on movies as their major method of presentation. Audio-visual materials must be carefully selected and previewed before their use in the classroom. Teacher and student demonstrations and problem-solving techniques tend to have long-lasting effects. In the final analysis, the effectiveness of a teaching method is shown in its lasting effects on the child, and its tendency to develop desirable behavior and to modify undesirable behavior.

In order to select the proper course content and teaching materials, one should understand the "processes" involved in developing safe behavior, which is the ultimate goal of safety education. Safe behavior is the optimum performance of a progression of seven dynamic processes:

1. Identification.
2. Assessment.
3. Decision.
4. Performance.
5. Evaluation.
6. Modification.
7. Application.[9]

This list explains what happens when a person is developing self-reliance and safe behavior. First, he "identifies" the hazards inherent in a given activity. He must understand how these relate to himself, to others, and to the environment. Then he "assesses" the risks in terms of his own mental, physical, and emotional capabilities, and in relation to others and to the environment. He "decides" which actions he must take to perform safely and which actions will allow the maximum fulfillment of his goals. He is then ready to "perform" in the safest possible manner.

After performance he must "evaluate" his actions and their outcome. He may then "modify" them in accordance with safe behavioral principles and try to make them even more safe, which may mean changing his

[9] National Safety Council, "Teaching About Safety," *Elementary Education Resource Unit*, Vol. I, ed. Susan Seder (Chicago, 1973), p. 3.

concept of what is and is not safe. He can then "apply" his experiences, knowledge, habits, and skills in a safe and meaningful manner to reach his desired goal.

It would be helpful in teaching safety to educate people to apply these processes with consistency. Figure 9-3 illustrates what is involved in developing safe behavior from the school standpoint.

SAFETY EDUCATION IN THE ELEMENTARY SCHOOL

The elementary school is the first opportunity to expose most children to planned safety education experiences. It should be the beginning of a positive approach to safety and safety education. For the first time children are being challenged with going to and from school. For the first time most of them are spending extended periods away from the immediate vicinity of their homes. They must learn to cross streets safely. They must form the habit of looking right, left, and right again before crossing. They must learn the meaning of traffic signs and signals.

The good elementary school teacher plans for safety education experiences that will meet the challenges facing children at this age. Safety education from kindergarten through the third grade will be handled largely by integrating it with other subjects. There are safety issues inherent in many lessons at the elementary level. The teacher should supervise closely at first and then gradually withdraw supervision as the children develop self-reliance and the ability to judge for themselves whether or not they are performing the assigned task in a safe manner.

Ideally, the teacher should precede the teaching of every new task by explaining the safe way to do it. For example, in crossing the street the teacher should say "This is the safe way to cross the street" instead of "Don't do it this way."

The primary emphasis at the elementary school level should be on the development of safe habits and skills. Children in this age group do not have long attention spans. Much repetition and practice will be necessary under the guidance and supervision of the teacher. Soon the children will start to identify and assess the inherent hazards on their own, a sign that they are beginning to understand.

Traffic safety is one of the most important aspects of safety education at the elementary level. Pedestrian and bicycle safety are integral parts of any good elementary school program. The development of safe behavior in play activities is also an important objective. Children should be encouraged to bring toys to school, and to analyze and discuss the

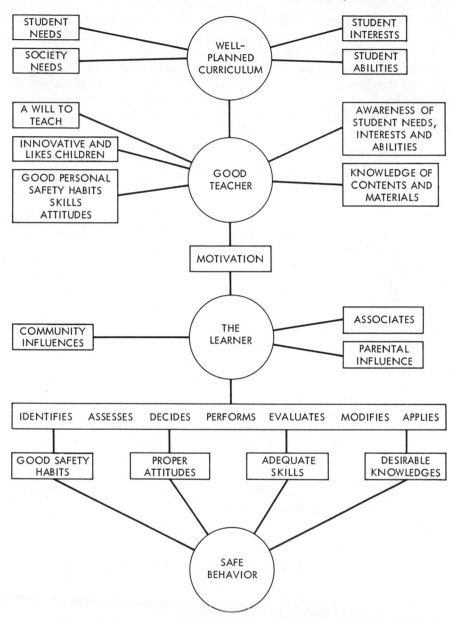

Figure 9-3. Developing safe behavior.

safe ways to use them and the hazards of using them unsafely. Reading can be taught by the use of stories related to safety. Safety education can be integrated into almost every subject at the elementary level.

The danger of teaching safety by integrating it with other subjects is that the teacher may not stress safety enough to develop the attitudes, skills, habits, and knowledge necessary for safe behavior. Most teacher-training institutions do not place enough emphasis on safety education. As a result teachers at all levels are generally unaware of the safety needs of their students. These same teachers often do not possess the necessary knowledge and skills to teach safety in a truly effective manner.

SAFETY EDUCATION IN THE JUNIOR HIGH SCHOOL

At this age the junior high school student is strengthening the attitudes he or she will carry throughout life. Major emphasis should be placed on the development of desirable attitudes toward safety. The fact that an interest in the opposite sex is increasing at this time makes the junior high school student susceptible to good safety attitudes. He or she should realize that acceptance by the opposite sex will depend to a large degree on good safe behavior. No one wants to associate with a person who consistently behaves in an unsafe manner.

Junior high students generally take health education as a separate subject. The objectives of these courses are almost, if not totally, identical with safety education. Most health education courses have separate units for safety education. Interest in cars, motor scooters, or the like increases at this age level, and represents opportunities for teaching safe behavior. Increased hazards in the physical activities of junior high school children are another opportunity for safety education. The emphasis should be on the development of good attitudes and the elimination of undesirable ones. Knowledge and understanding of safety rules and regulations also become more important.

SAFETY EDUCATION IN THE HIGH SCHOOL

The high school is the last chance for many children to experience formal, planned education. Since some students leave school after reaching sixteen, safety education courses should be given at the freshman and sophomore levels. Ironically, those who leave are probably the ones who need safety education the most. There is every indication that an educated person is a safer person.

integrating safety with school subjects

The most publicized safety course at the high school level is driver education. However, the well-planned safety education curriculum gives careful consideration to the opportunities for safety instruction inherent in other school subjects.

HEALTH. The goals of health and safety education are, for the most part, identical. First aid or common emergency situations and others are excellent opportunities for safety education experiences.

BIOLOGY. Much of the teaching in biology is directly related to health and safety education, such as the handling of plants and animals and the safety problems connected with them.

HOME ECONOMICS. The home economics teacher is concerned with safety aspects of food handling and cooking. A home economics course must deal with the safe use of the various appliances and utensils found in the kitchen. Safety must be a first consideration in such teaching.

INDUSTRIAL ARTS AND SHOPS. Safety in the handling of tools and equipment must be given priority. Every good shop teacher spends a considerable amount of time in direct safety teaching. He should begin teaching any new skill with the words, "This is the safe way to do this." His constant supervision of machine guards, his orderliness, and other factors help to make students safety minded.

CHEMISTRY AND PHYSICS. The handling of dangerous chemicals requires that the chemistry teacher include safety teaching in the normal routine. Many principles of accident prevention are learned in chemistry and physics labs. Practically all of the principles in physics have safety implications.

SOCIAL STUDIES. The study of courts, enforcement procedures, and laws can be related to safety. A visit to a court or other field trips have tremendous safety applications. Social studies teachers can add much to the development of good attitudes toward safety, especially in stressing the proper regard for traffic law enforcement.

MATHEMATICS. Safety and accident statistics make meaningful math exercises. Accident statistics are clearly relevant to students. Accident rates and trends are excellent resource material for mathematics classes and projects.

ENGLISH. Many safety education experiences can be strengthened by writing themes on different aspects of safety. It might be useful, for example, to assign themes on the problems of safety in recreation.

Safety can be correlated or integrated with any subject in the school curriculum. It calls for good planning to reduce overlap and to widen existing opportunities. Plans for the teaching of safety in all phases of the school program should be given the most careful consideration and promotion. No opportunity for safety education should be overlooked.

THE MODERN DRIVER EDUCATION PROGRAM

Modern driver education programs are divided into two phases—classroom instruction and laboratory instruction. The National Commission on Safety Education lists the following topics, not as a teaching outline, but as an indication of the nature and scope of content for a complete program in driver education. They are:

Traffic citizenship—responsibility to other drivers and highway users, community, family, or self; attitudes of safe living; courtesy and manners; support of public officials; traffic control devices.

Laws and regulations and their enforcement by courts—uniform traffic laws and ordinances; state motor vehicle laws; uniform vehicle code and model traffic ordinances; official safety agencies.

Characteristics of drivers—mental, emotional, physical, and physiological.

Society and driving—effects of alcohol and drugs; psychology and driving; our culture and driving.

Driving skills—basic habits and maneuvers; driving in the city, on the highway, on expressways; hazardous conditions and meeting emergencies; efficient driving.

Development of judgments—vision and perception; knowledge and analysis of traffic situations; making decisions; reaction time; physical laws that affect drivers and pedestrians.

The motor vehicle—history and development; economics of vehicle ownership; trip planning; mechanics of the vehicle; safety devices; vocational driving.

Traffic accidents—causes; human and economic loss; what to do in case of an accident; built-in response system for meeting the unexpected.

Engineering—automotive, highway, traffic.[10]

[10] National Education Association, *Driver and Traffic Safety Education* (Washington, D. C., 1964), pp. 4-5.

the classroom phase

Standard high school driver and traffic safety education courses should extend over a full semester (90 hours). If this is not feasible, a minimum of 30 class hours should be planned.[11]

One of the newer innovations in the classroom phase is called the drivocator system. It is an example of space-age electronics in the classroom. Students are equipped with responder units that allow them to respond to multiple choice questions shown on a screen. The responses register on the instructor's console. Figure 9-4 shows the drivocator system in operation.

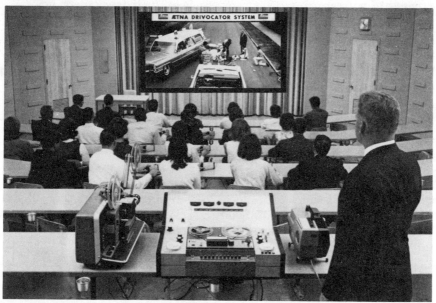

Figure 9-4. *A modern drivocator system, in use in many schools. Photo courtesy of Aetna Life and Casualty.*

Several excellent textbooks cover the topics suggested by the National Safety Commission. They are also compatible with the drivocator system.

the laboratory phase

The laboratory phase of driver education concerns behind-the-wheel experiences. Modern school programs approach this phase with a combination of methods:

[11] National Education Association, *Driver and Traffic Safety Education*, p. 22.

1. Simulation experience.
2. Multiple-car range experience.
3. In-traffic experience.

SIMULATOR EXPERIENCE. Simulators are another space-age electronic introduction in the classroom. This type of experience has been validated by research. The simulator systems incorporate all the motion controls and instruments found in conventional automobiles. This instruction method is particularly attractive and feasible because it allows more students to gain experience with fewer instructors and cars than would otherwise be possible. With the use of a movie screen, students are exposed to a great many driving experiences, including emergencies.

The instructor is equipped with a console that shows driving errors requiring immediate correction. Some consoles have permanent print-outs to provide a record of the student's progress.

The National Safety Commission suggests that if simulation experience is substituted for behind-the-wheel experience, it should be done on a ratio of a minimum of four hours of simulator experience for each hour of experience at the controls of a practice driving car. It recommends that credit for simulator experience not be counted for more than one-half of the school requirements for practice driving. It also recommends a minimum of six clock hours of laboratory experience.[12] Most schools today exceed this minimum requirement. Some states allow a certain amount of simulator time to be substituted for a portion of the minimum classroom time. However, they do not allow the same time in the simulator to be counted toward both classroom and practice driving time. Figure 9-5 shows a simulator classroom in operation.

MULTIPLE-CAR RANGE EXPERIENCE. The advantage of multiple-car range experience, which has also been validated through research, is that it reduces teacher-pupil ratios, just as simulators do. It permits several automobiles to be operated simultaneously under the direction of one or more teachers. This also has the advantage of being an off-street facility, allowing traffic conflict to be controlled by the instructor.

Some of the more sophisticated facilities have two-way radio contact between the instructor and the students. Figure 9-6 illustrates a modern range facility with a skid pan.

More schools are adding skid pans to their facilities today. Some skid pans are designed with an asphalt surface that becomes slippery when flooded. This gives the student an excellent opportunity to meet his or her first skidding situation under controlled conditions.

[12] National Education Association, *Driver and Traffic Safety Education*, p. 23.

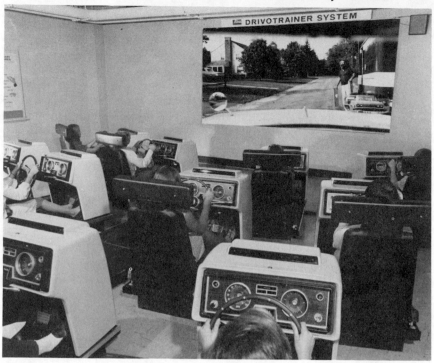

Figure 9-5. A simulator classroom. Photo courtesy of Aetna Life and Casualty.

IN-TRAFFIC EXPERIENCE. In the first driver education programs, the behind-the-wheel phase was actually started on the streets and, in

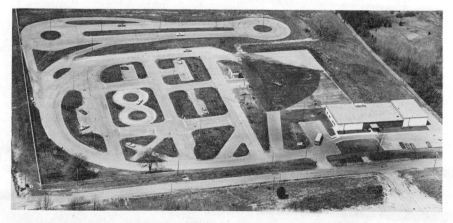

Figure 9-6. A well-designed driving range with a skid pan. Photo courtesy of Missouri Safety Center, Central Missouri State University.

many cases, in traffic. In most modern programs students are not exposed to in-traffic experience until they have progressed through classroom, simulation, and multiple-car experience on a driving range. As much time as possible should be allowed for in-traffic experience. The more advanced students should be shifted from the range to the in-traffic situation as soon as they are ready for the transition.

In-traffic experience should include city and highway driving in both day and night. Other students in the car can gain valuable experience just by observing the driver.

financing driver education programs

Driver education programs can be financed in many ways—by tuition, for example. Illinois, which has one of the best financed programs in the nation, adds an additional charge to every state driver's license fee. Since all drivers benefit from a program designed to educate younger drivers—an educated driver is a safer driver—the charge seems fair and equitable.

TASK ANALYSIS APPROACH TO DRIVING

Driving is a task that requires a type of social interdependence and interaction. It involves the thinking of millions of people.[13] The driving task includes observing, evaluating, and deciding how best to control the speed and position of the car for safe and efficient movement.[14] An error in this chain of events could result in an accident.

The driving task should be analyzed in light of what we know and understand about human behavior. This involves perception. The analysis should also give consideration to the automobile and the highway itself. Figure 9-7 illustrates the task analysis approach to driving.

This kind of approach is actually a type of systems analysis. It represents a problem-solving technique that can be followed in curriculum planning.[15]

Figure 9-8 illustrates two types of approaches to curriculum development. It shows the task analysis and the accident causation approaches. Present programs of driver education evolved from the accident causation approach.[16] However, the accident causation approach is too negative.

[13] *Driver Education for Illinois Youth* (Springfield, Ill.: The Office of the Superintendent of Public Instruction, 1972), p. 59.
[14] *Driver Education for Illinois Youth*, p. 59.
[15] *Driver Education for Illinois Youth*, p. 51.
[16] *Driver Education for Illinois Youth*, p. 51.

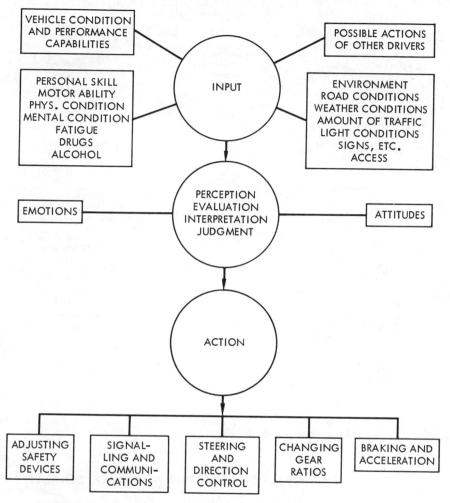

Figure 9-7. *An analysis of the driving task. Adapted from Driving Task Model,* Driver Education for Illinois Youth, *p. 59.*

The task analysis approach is positive; it gives more meaning to the curriculum and is more objective from the student's standpoint. It is recommended for the development of objectives for future driver education programs.

Regardless of the approach selected for curriculum development, one must consider the needs, interests, and comprehension abilities of the students. They should also have the opportunity to participate in the curriculum development process.

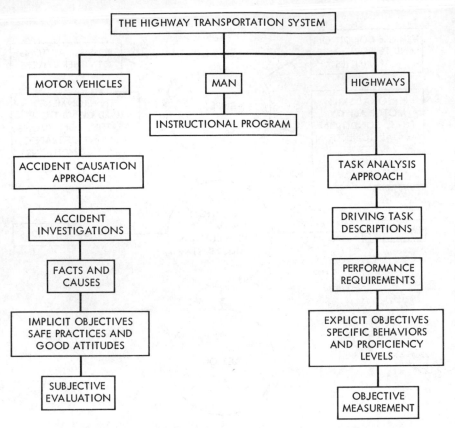

Figure 9-8. *Approaches for curriculum development. Adapted from* Driver Education for Illinois Youth, *p. 52.*

TEACHER PREPARATION IN DRIVER EDUCATION

Over the years the qualifications for teachers in driver education have constantly been upgraded. The National Commission on Safety Education of the NEA recommends the following: [17]

1. Introduction to Safety Education—3 sem. hours.
2. Driver and Traffic Safety—9 sem. hours.
3. Electives in the Behavior Sciences—3-6 sem. hours.

[17] National Education Association, *Driver and Traffic Safety Education,* pp. 12–13.

4. Electives dealing with legislation, enforcement, engineering, motor vehicle administration, community relations, and others—3-6 sem. hours.

This represents a minimum 18 semester-hour sequence. Figure 9-9 shows a task analysis of the teaching of driver education. Results of this analysis would indicate a definite need for additional courses in the following areas:

1. First aid and emergency procedures.
2. Health education courses.
3. A course to understand fully the interrelationships in our highway transportation system. It would deal with the problems of the auto design engineer and the problems of road design.
4. A course in instructional material.

Driver and traffic safety courses should include simulator experience, as well as range and behind-the-wheel teaching experience under the supervision of a well-trained staff.

SUMMARY

Schools must refine and upgrade their safety education curriculum. The development of desirable safety habits, attitudes, skills, and knowledge can make tremendous strides in accident prevention. The safety education curriculum must be constantly revised to keep pace with today's rapidly growing technology.

Schools must delegate the authority to well-qualified people and hold them accountable. The results of our driver education programs and of educational efforts in industry are direct evidence that good safety education pays dividends.

Teacher education institutions should upgrade their safety education training. The poor safety education backgrounds of many teachers result in a deemphasis of safety education at all school levels.

Schools hold a great potential for the development of safe and self-reliant people. They must place more emphasis on safety education. We cannot afford the "trade off" of human lives for a few minutes spent daily in the classroom on safety education.

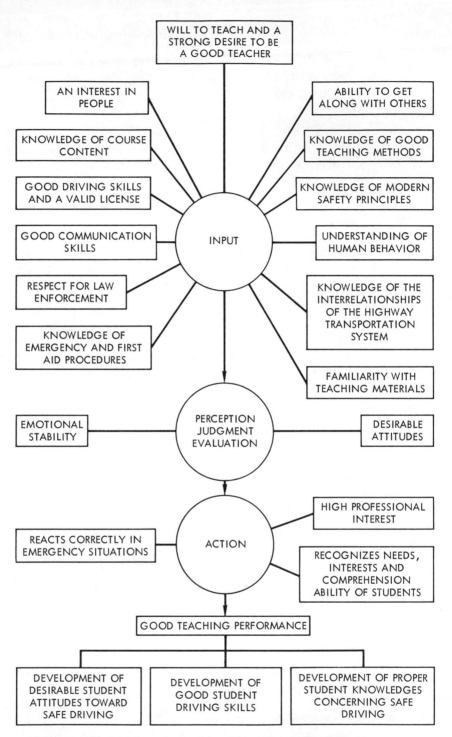

Figure 9-9. A task analysis of teaching driver education.

SUGGESTED STUDENT ACTIVITIES

1. Prepare a task analysis of a childhood activity.
2. Write a paper on the need for safety education in the school curriculum.
3. Survey your community and determine the voluntary and official agencies with school safety-related interests.
4. Write a definition of safety education.
5. List your daily activities and analyze the safety hazards connected with them.
6. Write five instructional objectives for a specified grade level and decide how you would measure the objectives.
7. Select two of the listed teaching methods and show how you would use them in a specified safety lesson.
8. Develop a lesson plan for a 50-minute safety lesson.
9. Develop a 6-week unit of safety instruction.
10. Develop a written plan for organizing an elementary school class into child-centered activities with the various groups working at their own speeds on different projects.

BIBLIOGRAPHY

AMERICAN ASSOCIATION OF SCHOOL ADMINISTRATORS. *Imperatives in Education.* Washington, D. C., 1966.

Driver Education for Illinois Youth. Springfield, Ill.: The Office of the Superintendent of Public Instruction, 1972.

KEY, NORMAN. "Safety Education." In *Curriculum Handbook for School Executives,* edited by Wm. J. Ellena. Washington, D.C.: American Association of School Administrators, 1973.

NATIONAL EDUCATION ASSOCIATION. *Driver and Traffic Safety Education.* Washington, D. C., 1964.

NATIONAL SAFETY COUNCIL. "Work Together." *Safety Education,* September 1960.

———. "Teaching About Safety," *Elementary Education Resource Unit,* Vol. I, edited by Susan Seder. Chicago, 1973.

NEAGLEY, ROSS L., and EVANS, N. DEAN. *Handbook for Effective Curriculum Development.* Englewood Cliffs, N. J.: Prentice-Hall, Inc., 1967.

STACK, HERBERT J., and ELKOW, J. DUKE. *Education for Safe Living.* 4th ed. Englewood Cliffs, N. J.: Prentice-Hall, Inc., 1966.

ZIRBES, LAURA. "How Shall We Teach Them Safety?" *School Safety* 4, No. 2, January-February 1969.

10

a safe school environment

The school's responsibility for the safety of its students begins when the children leave home for classes and does not end until they return. Therefore to create and maintain a safe school environment, one must not only consider the building and grounds but also the movement of students to and from school.

ACCIDENT RECORDS AND REPORTING SYSTEMS

The lack of accident records and reporting systems is one of the biggest weaknesses in school safety programs. This lack involves all areas of school safety. We do not have reliable statistics on accidents in school buses, buildings, or grounds, or on accidents in athletic programs.

It is impossible to make an accurate analysis of hazards or types of accidents without adequate data. Setting up good accident record systems is the first step in the organization of any safety program. Failure to complete an accident report form may be grounds for a lawsuit, since such a failure is considered negligence in itself. A centralized accident reporting system for each school system, as well as a similar national system, should be compulsory. Only then can we begin to make an accurate diagnosis of the accident situation as it exists in our schools today.

The accident record form should be detailed enough to give information that will aid remedial planning. Only when we make use of past accident experience can we begin to make more significant gains in accident prevention programs. Figure 10-1 is an example of a recommended accident report form.

(check one) ☐ School Jurisdictional ☐ Non-School Jurisdictional School District: City, State:	**RECOMMENDED** **STANDARD STUDENT ACCIDENT REPORT** (See instructions on reverse side)

General

1. Name			2. Address		
3. School		4. Sex Male ☐ Female ☐	5. Age	6. Grade/Special Program	
7. Time Accident Occurred Date:		Day of Week:		Exact Time:	AM ☐ PM ☐

Injury

8. Nature of Injury

9. Part of Body Injured

10. Degree of Injury (check one) Death ☐   Permanent ☐   Temporary (lost time) ☐   Non-Disabling (no lost time) ☐

11. Days Lost From School: From Activities Other Than School: Total:

12. Cause of Injury

Accident

13. Accident Jurisdiction (check one) School: Grounds ☐ Building ☐ To and From ☐ Other Activities Not on School Property ☐ Non-School: Home ☐ Other ☐

14. Location of Accident (be specific)

15. Activity of Person (be specific)

16. Status of Activity

17. Supervision (if yes, give title & name of supervisor) Yes ☐ No ☐

18. Agency Involved

19. Unsafe Act

20. Unsafe Mechanical/Physical Condition

21. Unsafe Personal Factor

22. Corrective Action Taken or Recommended

23. Property Damage School $ Non-School $ Total $

24. Description (Give a word picture of the accident, explaining who, what, when, why and how)

Signature

25. Date of Report

26. Report Prepared by (signature & title)

27. Principal's Signature

This form is recommended for securing data for accident prevention and safety education. School districts may reproduce this form adding space for optional data. Reference: Student Accident Reporting Guidebook. National Safety Council, 425 N. Michigan Avenue, Chicago, Illinois 60611. 1966. 34 pages.

Figure 10-1. *A student accident report form. Courtesy of the National Safety Council.*

PLANNING NEW SCHOOL FACILITIES

The planning of new school facilities should be part of the master planning process for the entire community. This long-range procedure requires extensive study and collection of data and involves the cooperation of many people and agencies. The school must fit into the total community pattern and be designed to meet as many particular community needs as possible.

Planning for the school should be closely coordinated with the recreational facilities in the community. Proper planning will allow the learning and teaching processes to extend into the community. The school is an ideal place for all community members to enjoy many physical, social, and intellectual pursuits.[1]

Higher and higher building costs are a serious concern, but safety cannot be sacrificed to economy. It must be the primary concern when planning a new facility, and the plans must be equally effective for the outside, as well as the inside.

site selection

Site selection is of vital importance in providing a safe school environment. The Council on Educational Facility Planners has established guidelines for minimum school site sizes, as follows:

Elementary schools—10 acres plus one acre per 100 students.
Junior high schools—20 acres plus one acre per 100 students.
Senior high schools—30 acres plus one acre per 100 students.[2]

These calculations should, of course, be based on ultimate rather than initial enrollments. The site's accessibility is of great importance since it will determine the distances to be traveled by the students. School-ground approaches must give consideration to pedestrian safety, bicycles, automobiles, and school buses. No hazardous crossroads should be nearby. Provision should be made for sidewalks and good roads. The site should be free of heavy traffic during opening and closing school hours.[3] Underpasses and pedestrian bridges should be used. These are

---

[1] Arthur H. Mittelstaedt, Jr., "Planning School Grounds," *Journal of Health, Physical Education and Recreation* 40, No. 5 (May 1969), p. 37.

[2] Nickolaus L. Engelhardt, *Complete Guide for Planning New Schools* (West Nyack, N. Y.: Parker Publishing Company, Inc., 1970), p. 264.

[3] Engelhardt, *Complete Guide for Planning New Schools*, p. 268.

only a few of the safety considerations in school site selection, but they do indicate the extensive planning that is necessary.

building design

The design of a school building should incorporate features that are conducive to safe movement, including adequate provisions for the handicapped, such as ramps instead of stairs. Special attention should be given to the widths of stairs, hallways, and exits. If hallways are too narrow, they become a safety hazard in the event of emergency evacuation. They also create traffic jams between classes.

All new buildings should be designed so that special hazards can be separated from other areas. Shops, chemistry laboratories, boiler rooms, supply rooms, and others have special hazards inherent in them.[4] Of all the safety hazards in such rooms, fire is the biggest problem. Ideally these rooms should be located so that fire cannot spread rapidly from them to other parts of the building. In larger school systems it may be feasible to locate the more fire-susceptible rooms in separate buildings.[5]

All building areas should be constructed of fire-resistant materials. The degree of resistance should, of course, be in line with existing building codes and the intended use of the room. Rooms with special hazards should be equipped with automatic fire detection systems and automatic sprinklers.

Figure 10-2 shows a high-speed water deluge fire protective system. The goal in this system is the fast cooling of the combustion process. The total distribution of the extinguishing agent in the primary suppression and the total activation of the backup deluge system is accomplished in milliseconds. High-speed thermocouples are used to sense over-temperature and actuate the system.

Even though a building may be virtually fireproof in construction, it is impossible to furnish it with completely fire-resistant contents. Since schools contain large amounts of paper and other combustibles, they will always have a degree of fire susceptibility.

Adequate alarm systems should be installed with backup systems. Both manual and automatic fire alarm systems should be installed.

The building should have an adequate and reliable system for reporting fires. Preferably the fire alarm system should be connected directly to the fire department. In the future sophisticated devices such

[4] Chester I. Babcock and Rexford Wilson, *The Chicago School Fire* (Boston: National Fire Protection Association, 1959), p. 24.
[5] Babcock and Wilson, *Chicago School Fire*, p. 24.

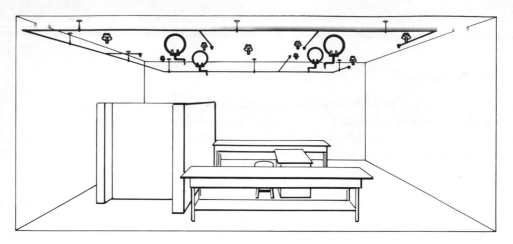

Figure 10-2. A room with a high-speed water deluge fire protection system. Courtesy of Fenwal, Inc., Protective Systems Division, Ashland, Mass.

as electronic boards in fire stations will not only show when a school is on fire, but will mark the particular room that is affected.

Heating and air conditioning systems should be installed with great care. Systems designed to circulate air throughout a building may also provide an avenue for the rapid spread of fire and smoke.[6]

Maintenance and good housekeeping are big factors in safety and fire prevention. Possible maintenance problems should be considered during the planning stages of construction. Proper color guards and symbols should be placed throughout the building to signify the different types of hazards. Good maintenance pays for itself in the long run. It is important both from the standpoint of safety and economy. There is no excuse for any school system to tolerate poor maintenance.

EXISTING SCHOOL BUILDINGS

Good master planning takes into consideration older existing buildings, not only plans for new facilities. All school buildings, new or old, must meet the highest safety standards.

A deep concern for safety in school buildings is surely warranted, for an estimated 15,000 school fires occur annually in the United States. Fortunately, few of them represent immediate danger to students. How-

[6] Babcock and Wilson, *Chicago School Fire*, p. 25.

ever, the danger inherent in fires is always present and should never be underestimated.[7]

Several cases of disastrous school fires in past years are grim evidence of those facts. In 1908 a school fire in Ohio killed 175 people. In 1936 a Texas school explosion and fire took 294 lives. In 1958, 90 students and 3 teachers died in a school fire in Chicago; 77 others were seriously injured.[8] More recently there have been 31 public-school fires with a reported loss of over $250,000 each. These catastrophes show the need for precaution regarding potential school fires.[9]

Unfortunately, a large number of school buildings in use today in the United States are not really fire safe. Remodeling a building is a costly and time-consuming process. In many cases the cost of remodeling old buildings to make them meet existing building codes may approach the cost of new construction. A careful analysis of an old building should be made before extensive remodeling is begun. What a waste to spend thousands of dollars on an old school and still end up with a building that has a short life expectancy.

Certain conditions do warrant either immediate correction or the discontinued use of an existing building until such time as the conditions are corrected. Past school fires clearly indicate that the following conditions should be corrected immediately:

1. Buildings where the walls or ceilings of exit corridors are surfaced with highly combustible finishes.
2. Buildings with wood floors and masonry walls, especially if the pupils in the upper floors have no means of exit other than through stairs open to lower stories.
3. Buildings of wood construction with pupils housed above the second story.
4. Buildings with unventilated space below them. Gas collects in these spaces and may explode.
5. Buildings with exit doors to the outside that cannot be readily opened from the inside.
6. Buildings in which pupils on upper floors have no means of exit except down stairs which are open to lower stories having combustible walls and finishes or contents in storage which are combustible.[10]

Buildings with inadequate electrical circuits for today's modern electrical equipment in classrooms and media centers present a real fire

---

[7] National Safety Council, *School Fire Safety*, Safety Education Data Sheet No. 47 rev. (Chicago, n.d.).

[8] National Fire Protection Association, *Occupancy Fire Record*, Fire Record FR 57-1A (Boston, 1965), pp. 17–18.

[9] National Safety Council, *School Fire Safety*.

[10] American Insurance Association, *Safe Schools* (New York, 1968), p. 4.

hazard. Additional circuitry with sufficient outlets in appropriate places is needed.

All older buildings should be carefully analyzed for potential safety hazards. Safety education classes should be instructed to make such an analysis.

SCHOOL GROUNDS

A recent report by the National Safety Council showed that of all the school jurisdictional accidents, 50 percent were on school grounds.[11] There are, however, no adequate statistics available on deaths and injuries resulting from playground accidents. Some of the general principles or guidelines for the safe use of play areas on the school grounds are:

1. Segregate the activities. Areas for small children should be marked off from other areas.
2. Paths should lead from the entrances to the main center of interest.
3. Color codes should be used to aid the children. Use of high-

[11] National Safety Council, *Play Areas*, Safety Education Data Sheet No. 29 (Chicago, n.d.).

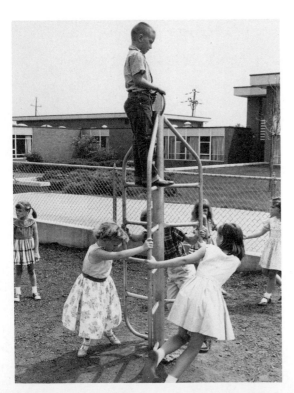

Figure 10-3. *A well-designed school playground. Note how the jungle gym is separated from other activities. Photo courtesy of the National Safety Council.*

visibility yellow for slide steps, edges of teeter boards, swing seats, and other areas is suggested. Fire protection equipment should be red. White lines should show boundary lines.

4. Apparatus should be concentrated in one area rather than scattered.
5. Age groupings should be considered in the placement of apparatus.
6. Rules should be prominently posted.
7. Apparatus should never be placed close to game fields.
8. Swings should be set in concrete and thoroughly tested. Swing seats should have bumper protectors.
9. Swings should be set at different heights for different age groups.
10. Slides should be placed in the shade if possible since the chutes become hot after standing in the sun.
11. Sand or sand and sawdust should be placed at the bottom of the slide, replaced at regular intervals, and kept clean.
12. Teeter board fulcrums should be protected to prevent catching fingers near the center of the board.
13. Children should be instructed in the use of teeter boards, and the rules enforced.
14. Only small children should use sandboxes, and they should be checked frequently for broken glass and other debris.
15. Drinking fountains should be kept free from rubbish and in accordance with health department regulations.[12]

This is only a partial list of the many guidelines that should be used to promote safety on playgrounds and related areas.

Every school should develop its own rules and regulations. Playgrounds should be closely supervised. Most states have regulations concerning the student–supervisor ratios for playground safety.

Parking lots should meet existing state and federal standards. Special attention should be given to the circulation of traffic and the widths of the parking spaces. A well-designed lot will ease parking problems and reduce many unnecessary accidents. Exits and entrances should be designed to reduce traffic hazards from the companion roadways.

TO AND FROM SCHOOL

The movement of children to and from school is accomplished in several different ways. Schools are involved in the following ways:

[12] National Safety Council, *Play Areas.*

1. Providing school safety patrols.
2. Providing school bus transportation.
3. Controlling traffic problems in and around the school grounds generated by students operating their own vehicles or being driven to school by someone else.
4. Planning desirable routes for students walking to and from school.

school safety patrols

School safety patrols, a key force in protecting our nation's children, date back to the early 1920's. Over 20 foreign countries now also use school safety patrols.[13] Millions of youngsters over the years have served in these organizations, and today the same work is carried on by their children.[14] Recognized as a national institution, the school safety patrol is a respected element in accident prevention. Much credit must go to the American Automobile Association and its affiliated clubs for their great contribution to the organization and promotion of these patrols.

FUNCTIONS OF SCHOOL SAFETY PATROLS. Although they may be utilized in different ways, such as hall guards, school safety patrols have two basic functions. They are: [15]

1. To instruct, direct, and control the members of the student body in crossing streets and highways at or near the schools.
2. To assist teachers and parents in the instruction of school children in safe pedestrian practices at all times.

It is not the function of school safety patrols to direct vehicular traffic in and around schools, nor should they be allowed to function in such a manner.[16]

ORGANIZATION OF SCHOOL SAFETY PATROLS. The school administration, with school board approval, is responsible for organizing school safety patrols. Several factors determine the patterns that are used. The administration of school safety patrols is similar to that of other phases of school administration. Policies are usually determined by committees under the direction of the superintendent and principals. The direct supervision of the patrols is usually placed in the hands of a competent and interested teacher. The teacher-supervisor is the key person in the

[13] American Automobile Association, *How to Organize a School Safety Patrol* (Washington, D. C., 1960), p. 3.
[14] American Automobile Association, *School Safety Patrol*, p. 3.
[15] American Automobile Association, *School Safety Patrol*, p. 69.
[16] American Automobile Association, *School Safety Patrol*, p. 69.

organization since his or her enthusiasm will keep the patrol members eager and willing to do a good job. Under the teacher or adult supervisor are the patrol officers, usually called captains and lieutenants. Figure 10-4 illustrates a typical organizational plan for a school safety patrol.

SELECTION OF PATROL MEMBERS. Different methods may be used for selecting patrol members, depending on the school and its policies. Some suggested ways of selection are: [17]

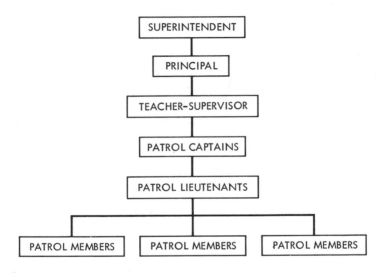

Figure 10-4. An organizational chart for a school safety patrol.

1. On a volunteer basis.
2. On a volunteer basis, then choosing the best volunteers by practical examinations in the safety rules that apply to patrol members.
3. Essays or the like to judge the knowledge of the safety rules involved.
4. Selection on the basis of the child's safety record at school.

Some suggested criteria for selection of patrol members are:

1. An interest in traffic safety.
2. Leadership ability.
3. Good judgment.
4. Desire to serve others.

[17] Chicago Motor Club, *School Safety Patrol Supervisors Manual* (Chicago, n.d.), p. 3.

5. Respect of classmates.
6. Punctuality.
7. Courtesy.
8. Good attendance records.
9. Reliability.
10. Will not exceed authority.[18]

ROUTES TO AND FROM SCHOOL. Large pin maps that show the location of the school population aid in the selection of the safest and best routes to and from school. These maps show intersections for converging points that are already equipped with traffic signals, and they also indicate the most direct routes. Parents as well as children should be informed of the best and safest routes to school. One parent should first walk the route with the child and instruct him or her in the use of the map.[19]

Physical characteristics and traffic conditions affect pedestrian safety along the route. Some examples of the things that should be considered are:

1. Availability of sidewalks. Use streets with sidewalks if possible.
2. Visibility at the various street crossings must be considered. Parking controls may be indicated.
3. Streets with frequent conflicts between pedestrians and vehicles should be avoided. (Heavy traffic over sidewalks.) [20]

Figure 10-5 illustrates a school safety patrol in action.

CLASSIFICATION OF CROSSWALKS. Classifying crosswalks involves the use of traffic counts and surveys. The amount of traffic at a particular crosswalk will determine whether a police officer, an adult guard, a safety patrol member, or some combination of the three should be used. Crosswalks are usually classified into three categories, as follows:

1. Those intersected by less than 120 vehicles per hour.
2. Those with over 120 but less than 300 vehicles per hour.
3. Those with over 300 vehicles per hour.[21]

At crosswalks intersected by less than 120 cars per hour, there usually is little need for protection since there are many gaps in traffic.

[18] Chicago Motor Club, *School Safety Patrol Supervisors Manual*, p. 8.
[19] Automotive Safety Foundation, *Guide to School Pedestrian Safety Program* (Washington, D. C., 1965), p. 10.
[20] Automotive Safety Foundation, *Pedestrian Safety Program*, p. 11.
[21] Automotive Safety Foundation, *Pedestrian Safety Program*, p. 4.

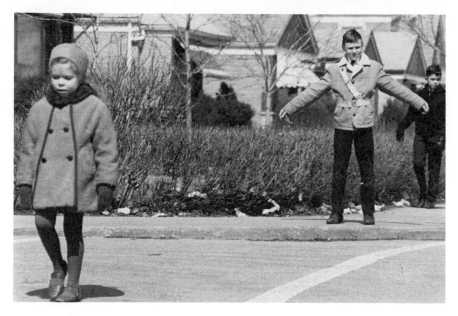

Figure 10-5. A school safety patrol in action. Photo courtesy of Chicago Motor Club, Patrol News.

These intersections do provide valuable training places for children. At crosswalks with traffic intersected by between 120 and 300 cars per hour, there are fewer gaps in the traffic and the hazards are increased. Patrols are especially valuable here in protecting children and providing a type of education that is vital to youngsters at this age. After the traffic count reaches 300 cars per hour at a crosswalk, a survey will determine if there are gaps in traffic. It is usually necessary to create gaps—using policemen, traffic lights, or stop signs—after traffic reaches 350 vehicles per hour.[22]

A traffic engineering department, if the city has one, can be most helpful in determining the proper method of creating gaps in the traffic. If there is no traffic engineering department, the police department should be consulted.

school bus transportation

School bus transportation adds greatly to the complexity of our highway transportation system. Although the school bus system does not appear large because it is broken down into small independent units,

[22] Automotive Safety Foundation, *Pedestrian Safety Program,* p. 5.

there are actually more than 300,000 school buses transporting over 20,000,000 pupils to and from school on a daily basis in this country. In a recent year there were approximately 45,000 school bus accidents, injuring some 6,000 people, 4,500 of whom were students.[23] In the same year about 180 deaths resulted from school bus transportation, including 100 pupils, 10 bus drivers, and 70 other people. Thirty-five of the pupils were passengers on school buses; 65 were pedestrians either approaching or leaving a loading zone. Over one-half of the pupil pedestrians were struck by a vehicle other than the school bus they were entering or leaving.[24]

Despite these figures, school bus transportation is a safe operation considering the number of children being transported, the number of school buses in use, and the number of miles driven. It should also be noted that about 90 percent of the accidents involved property damage but no personal injuries.

We must have well-planned and well-executed safety programs for school bus transportation. The responsibility for such programs lies with the individual school districts. Safety of the children should be the first consideration; economy, although important, must be secondary.

Each school district should have written policies, rules, and regulations to govern the operation of the school transportation system.[25] The school district should exercise supervision over the program within the framework of these established policies.[26]

With the enactment of the 1966 National Traffic and Motor Vehicle Act, the federal government has authority over school bus standards in each state.

STATE GUIDELINES FOR SCHOOL BUS SAFETY. The National Safety Council recommends the following guidelines for school bus safety:

1. Standards must be established for buses and equipment. They should go beyond the national guidelines, if necessary.
2. Maintenance standards should be set and enforced by competent personnel to insure that vehicles are maintained in safe operating condition. Superficial inspections by untrained personnel on a yearly basis will not satisfy this requirement.
3. Driver qualifications should be established. They should include mental and physical standards and strict licensing procedures.
4. Basic driver training programs should be provided, with mandatory attendance by drivers. This should include annual training schools or workshop sessions.

[23] National Safety Council, *Accident Facts 1973 Edition* (Chicago, 1973), p. 93.
[24] National Safety Council, *Accident Facts 1973*, p. 92.
[25] Paul T. Stewart, "The School and Pupil Transportation," *Traffic Safety*, July 1969, p. 12.
[26] Stewart, "The School and Pupil Transportation," p. 12.

5. Basic rules and regulations governing the transportation of pupils should be in effect. These should indicate the extent of the transportation services to be provided, the authority at various levels, and the expected behavior of the pupils. Privileges should be contingent upon behavior.
6. These minimums should apply to all school transportation in the state: public, non-public, school-owned or contracted.
7. The leadership at the state level should be extended to provide liaison among the departments of public instruction, public safety, motor vehicles, and state highway.
8. Personnel and funds should be made available to implement and provide for supervisory and inspection programs.
9. Another important function at the state level is the provision for adequate training facilities, seminars, and specialized courses to be offered for the different levels of responsibility.[27]

Uniform regulations covering school bus transportation should be adopted across the country. More complete accident records kept on a uniform basis will provide insights into methods for reducing school bus accidents. Figure 10-6 shows a school bus unloading passengers.

[27] National Safety Council, *School Transportation: A Guide for Supervisors* (Chicago, 1967), pp. 5–6.

Figure 10-6. A school bus unloading passengers. Photo courtesy of the National Safety Council.

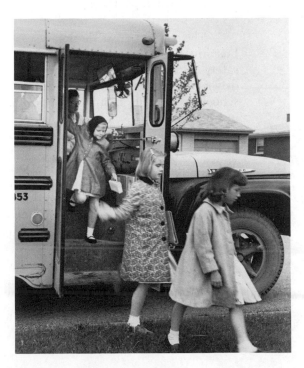

PROVIDING SAFE VEHICLES. Safe pupil transportation starts with the selection and use of safe vehicles. All buses in school service at any given time should meet or exceed the national, as well as the state, standards. Maintenance and inspection should be conducted on a regular basis by trained individuals. Good maintenance will not only reduce accidents, but will enable the buses to operate more economically. The school bus driver should faithfully check such things as horns, lights, brakes, and tires on a daily basis. A complete checklist for drivers should be furnished by the school system.

SELECTION OF THE DRIVER. The National Safety Council recommends the following considerations for driver selection.

1. Top physical fitness.
2. Honesty, punctuality, and dependability.
3. Good adjustment and emotional stability.
4. Size and stature to fit the job.
5. Impeccable references.
6. A congenial personality.
7. Acceptable driving skill or capacity for being trained.
8. No previous record of repeated traffic violations or preventable vehicular accidents.
9. Stable marital status.
10. Neat appearance.[28]

The state of West Virginia uses excellent procedures to select school bus drivers. They are required to pass a rigorous physical exam, a written safety test, and a check on criminal, credit, and military records. The drivers must take a 12-hour training program covering motor vehicle and school laws, pupil discipline, safe driving practices, and behind-the-wheel instruction.[29]

When hired, West Virginia school bus drivers must be over 21 and under 51. Once hired, they can drive until the mandatory retirement age of 65. After 50 they must have physical examinations twice a year and electrocardiograms once a year. All drivers must take a refresher course prior to the opening of each new school term.[30]

The proper selection of school bus drivers, coupled with proper training and supervision, is an important part of the total school transportation safety program.

[28] National Safety Council, *School Transportation*, p. 21.
[29] R. W. Crosby and V. Block, "How Safe Is the Ride to School?" *Traffic Safety*, October 1968, p. 13.
[30] Crosby and Block, "How Safe Is the Ride?" p. 13.

SCHOOL BUS PASSENGERS. The responsibility for educating school bus passengers is shared by the classroom teacher, the bus driver, the school administrator, and the parents. The students themselves must assume some of the responsibility for their education and safety while school bus passengers. They should be given every opportunity to acquire the necessary information and attitudes necessary for their safety.[31] Their personal conduct is of great importance.

These are some guiding principles regarding pupil safety and education:

1. Students should leave their homes in time to reach the bus loading site. They should know when the bus is scheduled to arrive.
2. Students walking along roads without sidewalks should walk on the left side facing traffic.
3. When boarding the bus they should always use the hand rail. They should board immediately when the bus arrives. No crowding or pushing should be allowed. Younger children should board first. Boys should let girls go first.
4. They should take their seats immediately and remain seated throughout the entire trip.
5. There are different methods used for children after they have alighted from the bus. Their instruction in these procedures should be thorough.
6. Instruction during the year should be varied and repeated as often as student conduct indicates a need for it.
7. There should be emphasis on self-reliance so that the student learns to accept responsibility for his own safety and becomes more safe.[32]

These are but a few of the things to be considered in student passenger education. Different localities have different problems. Education should deal with the specific problems in each locality.

STUDENT CONDUCT ON THE BUS. Student conduct on school buses should equal that in the classroom. The driver should have the same authority over the passenger as does the classroom teacher. Noise generated by passengers should be held to a minimum. It is said that in the future many buses will be equipped with television so that the student will be learning while on the bus. This should reduce the noise factor. Privileges and restrictions should be consistent with behavior,

[31] National Safety Council, *School Bus Passengers Safety,* Safety Education Data Sheet No. 63 (Chicago, n.d.).
[32] National Safety Council, *School Bus Passengers Safety.*

and sensible, fair rules should be enforced by the driver with school administration approval and backing.

EMERGENCY PROCEDURES. Both routine and emergency safety procedures should be taught to student passengers. Drills should be conducted so that the students know and understand the safe procedures for exiting under emergency conditions. They should know the location of emergency exits and how to operate them, including doors as well as windows. Figure 10-7 shows a school bus emergency drill.

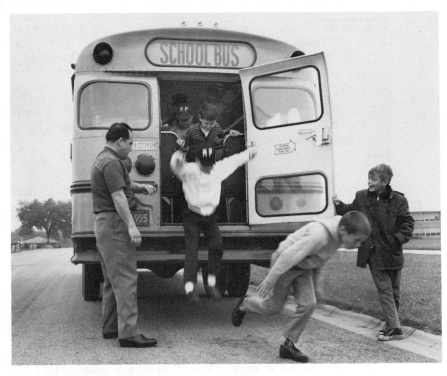

Figure 10-7. An emergency school bus drill. Photo courtesy of the National Safety Council.

STUDENT BUS PATROLS. Many schools use student bus patrols as part of their school bus safety programs. Sometimes these patrols are extensions of the school safety patrols.

Two students should be selected. Ideally they should live at the end of the route so that they will be on the bus for the longest period of time. They can help younger children on and off the bus safely, help the driver maintain order, and help students cross the streets and highways. One state even trained selected patrol members in how to stop the bus in case something incapacitated the driver. Taking attendance is another way the students can help.[33] They should be assigned duties that help the driver and make his work safer.

EXTENDED USE OF SCHOOL BUSES. Most communities use their school buses not only to transport children to and from school but also for such other activities as student field trips or athletic contests. When school buses are used in this manner, routes and speeds should be carefully selected. Such activities sometimes require the drivers to drive in unfamiliar places, thus increasing the danger of accidents. Another adult should supervise these trips.

traffic in and around school

Extra traffic is created around many schools by parents and others transporting children to and from school in private automobiles. If this becomes hazardous, steps must be taken to regulate loading and unloading sites and to give general directions to the traffic. Police departments should be asked to handle this problem. Another traffic problem often arises because students themselves drive to and from school. This traffic must be firmly regulated. Speed limits on the school grounds and parking regulations should be strictly enforced.

STUDENT TRAFFIC COURTS. A student traffic court in high school is an excellent way to promote self-regulation by the students. This method tends to foster the cooperation of all students. Most of these courts originate in student councils, but faculty supervision is needed because such courts have a tendency to become overly severe. The responsibilities and limits of authority of student courts must be delineated, and their valid decisions backed up by school administrators. Student traffic courts provide excellent learning experiences, and serve as a good control of student drivers.

SCHOOL EMERGENCY PREPAREDNESS

Every school should have a program of emergency preparedness that will meet the needs of its particular district and community. Many schools still have plans that are poorly organized, not in written form, and that, in case of an emergency, would be poorly executed. Emergency preparedness plans are like insurance. You may feel them to be unnecessary, but if and when you need them, you will need them badly.

[33] National Safety Council, *School Bus Passengers Safety.*

No school should be caught in an emergency situation without a well-organized plan that can be put into effect immediately and executed with smoothness and maximum efficiency. Anything less in the way of planning is gross negligence.

Negligence can and does happen, as has been dramatically illustrated many times during tornado, hurricane, or cyclone threats. School officials were hesitant and uncertain in their actions because they had no prearranged plans. Lack of planning creates panic. Panic aggravates an already serious situation and may in fact turn the situation into an unnecessary disaster.

Several areas should be considered in planning for emergency situations. Some of them are:

1. School crises such as riots.
2. Bomb threats.
3. School bus emergencies.
4. Civil defense.
5. Epidemics.
6. Crowd control at athletic events.
7. Chemical transportation and storage.
8. Building elevators.
9. Interruption of power services such as gas and lights.
10. Injury situations in gymnasiums, playgrounds, shops, and laboratories.
11. Fires.[34]

All possible emergencies in the community must be considered when preparing a workable plan. Planning committees should seek help from proper agencies in the community, such as fire departments, police departments, and civil defense units.

principles of emergency planning in schools

The following principles may be helpful in planning for school emergencies. Others should be added when applicable to each local situation.

1. The school board should authorize the school administration to prepare a plan for the board's adoption.
2. The school administration should appoint a person, preferably

[34] National Safety Council, *School Emergency Procedures for Emergencies of Man Made Origin*, Safety Education Data Sheet No. 36 (Chicago, n.d.).

the director of safety, to follow through on the planning and to be held accountable for the plan's development.

3. A committee should be assigned to guide the school system in the planning. It should have representation from appropriate community organizations, such as the fire department, police department, and civil defense agencies.

4. Provisions should be made for adequate budgeting, for development of the plan, and for its ultimate operation.

5. Uniform, systematic drills should be set up and carried out for the types of emergencies thought possible in that particular community.

6. The plan should be coordinated with any emergency plans for the community.

7. A system must be set up to inform students, teachers, administrators, and other school employees of all details of the plan.

8. Plans and policies should be in writing and strictly adhered to.

9. The plan should be compatible with federal, state, and local regulations.

10. Adequate provisions should be made for evacuation of the handicapped under emergency situations.

11. Areas having peculiar types of construction should be noted.

12. Communication procedures should be established, including plans for alternate procedures in the event that the primary communication system fails.

13. Planning should include special events such as athletic contests or school plays, where large groups may be concentrated in a specific area.

14. Plans should include emergency first aid procedures.

15. A system should be set up for evaluating and upgrading the plan on a periodic basis.

16. An adequate system of communication both for indoors and outdoors should be provided. Special fire alarm signals should be devised in cases of communication systems failures.

emergency fire drills

Emergency fire drills, when properly directed and executed, are excellent and necessary educational experiences. They help to prevent panic, and they set patterns of action for any future emergencies that may arise.

Some of the principles and characteristics of a good emergency drill and related precautions are the following:

1. Emergency drill regulations should be prepared specifically for each building within a school system.
2. Explicit directions should be posted in each room at a point where everyone can see them. Alternate routes should be indicated.
3. Special precautions should be taken for assembly rooms, lunchrooms, and other areas where there are large concentrations of people at any given time.
4. Teachers should be provided with written instructions on the handling of emergencies, including instructions on how to report a fire and special duties during a drill or fire.
5. Special attention should be given to areas with such things as power tools or heating equipment.
6. Teachers should be responsible for prompt sounding of the alarm or immediate notification of the principal's office (or both) in event of fire.
7. A fire should be reported *first*, before portable fire extinguishers are used. All teachers should know how to use fire extinguishers.
8. The duties and responsibilities of administrators should be written out.
9. All instructions should be reviewed with the local fire department.
10. Drill routines should be worked out with the best technical advice available. A representative of the fire department should attend the fire drills periodically to offer suggestions if necessary.
11. Emphasis should be on prompt response, not speed. Running should not be permitted.
12. Students should not be allowed to stop for coats. It is not necessary to call fire drills in bad weather.
13. Silence is important. Students should know the meaning of hand signals. Discipline and orderliness are imperative.
14. Different exits should be blocked during the drills to simulate emergency situations.
15. Drill routines should be written out and circulated so that all students understand them.
16. The written routines should be revised when necessary.
17. Teachers should take attendance records with them during the drill and take attendance immediately after they have safely cleared the building.
18. Schools should meet federal and state regulations concerning the suggested number of drills. Most states require one per month.

19. Fire alarm systems should have backup or alternate methods of notification in case the primary alarm system fails. They should meet state and local regulations and be approved by the Underwriters Laboratories.
20. No one should be allowed to reenter the building until a signal is given that it is safe to do so.
21. Records should be kept noting such things as the time required to clear the building. Any malfunctions in drill procedures should receive immediate attention.
22. Any detection of smoke should be immediately reported.
23. Students should know the proper methods of exit if forced to go through areas containing smoke.

Careful planning and practice of the plan is the best defense against possible injury in the event of fire or any other emergency. Every fire alert and drill should be treated seriously by everybody.[35]

SAFETY IN SPORTS AND PHYSICAL EDUCATION

Sports and physical education activities are fun and exciting. They challenge and stimulate people. They provide needed emotional and physical outlets, which enhance the mental, physical, and social well-being of the participants. These activities foster and promote competitive spirit. Sports and physical education make significant contributions to the total education program.

Most people will engage in some type of sport or exercise activity throughout most of their lives. Sports and physical education programs in the schools should develop the habits, attitudes, knowledge, and skills necessary for safe participation in various activities during later life.

Since many physical activities involve speed, vigorous exercise, quick movements, and body contact, the risk factor is higher than that found in the ordinary classroom situation. It is therefore not surprising that accidents and injuries on playgrounds, athletic fields, and in gymnasiums account for a major portion of the total accidents and injuries occurring in our schools.

Maximum enjoyment and fulfillment from sports and physical education can be attained only through safe and efficient participation. Accidents and injuries tend to defeat the purposes of the programs.

There is, of course, a calculated risk involved in sports and physical

[35] Most of these recommendations were taken from National Safety Council, *School Fire Safety.*

education activities. The amount of risk depends on many things—the physical condition of the participant, exposure or the amount of time spent in the activity, the nature of the activity itself, and the conditions under which the person engages in the activity.

Swimming, for example, could be considered a very dangerous activity under certain circumstances, but if done properly under controlled conditions it is very safe. Football, because of the amount of body contact under high speed conditions, could be dangerous. But under the right conditions, with proper equipment and supervision, thousands of people play football in relative safety.

The risk factor, then, is directly related to the specific variables inherent in the activity, the conditions, and the amount of exposure. Risk can and should be minimized by proper controls and precautions. Then the advantages of participation will usually outweigh any disadvantages.

programming for safety in sports and physical education

Like any other phase of accident prevention, safety in sports and physical education requires planning and careful execution of the plan. Risk can be significantly reduced by applying the following principles:

1. Recognition of the hazards present.
2. Removal of the hazards when possible.
3. Control over those hazards that cannot be removed.
4. The creation of no additional hazards.[36]

RECOGNITION OF HAZARDS. You must understand an activity in order to analyze the hazards inherent in it. You must also understand human characteristics as they relate to the activity, and you must know the environmental factors connected with the sport.

Once the hazards of an activity are recognized, the next step is an appropriate physical examination. It should determine to what extent, if any, an individual can participate safely. Certain health defects, such as poor vision or a circulatory condition, may limit participation or even preclude it altogether.

Height, weight, strength, endurance, coordination, motor ability, and other factors may make it hazardous for an individual to participate in a certain activity. These limits should help to determine the type of activity that an individual should seek. The individual's skill level may

[36] American Association for Health, Physical Education and Recreation, *School Safety Policies with Emphasis on Physical Education, Athletics and Recreation* (Washington, D. C., 1968), p. 8.

present certain additional hazards. Obviously skill level is very important in such activities as swimming or horseback riding. It also may largely determine the amount and type of supervision needed.

Recognizing hazards requires a thorough analysis of the environment where the activity takes place, the equipment, and the facility itself. Coaches, teachers, and other officials should make daily inspections of areas where students engage in physical activities. Wet grounds, for example, may rule out an athletic contest.

Recognition of the hazards enables the people involved to determine whether or not that hazard can be removed, controlled, or otherwise dealt with. If it cannot be removed, other action must be taken to limit the risks.

The task analysis approach by coaches and players would expose the hazards of many activities. It also indicates the special skills needed for performance of any activity.

REMOVAL OF HAZARDS. Once a hazard is exposed, if possible it should be removed immediately. Defective equipment, trash, or cut glass on or around playing surfaces are hazards that can be effectively controlled. Athletic fields, playgrounds, and gymnasiums should be designed to minimize conflict with other activities.

Planning will eliminate the hazards of unequal competition, length, and number of events. Too much competition in a specified period can be dangerous, a fact that should be considered in the structuring and timing of tournament play. Fatigue is often a triggering factor in athletic injuries. Proper physical conditioning helps to remove the hazards of fatigue.

There is no excuse for allowing people to engage in activities on slippery floors or under other hazardous conditions. Good maintenance of both the facility and the equipment plays a large role in removing or eliminating hazards, thus reducing or minimizing the chances of accident or injury.

CONTROL OF HAZARDS THAT CANNOT BE REMOVED. Hazards that cannot be removed should be controlled. For example, a wall at one end of an arena where players run at high speeds might be covered with mats to avoid injury. Swimming pools may need additional safety measures, especially when many people are in or around the water. Proper instruction concerning a specific hazard and good physical conditioning are other examples of hazard control.

Coaches and officials associations constantly strive to find rules that will promote safety. Certain game rules may have to be modified to accommodate certain facilities. Commonly known as ground rules, they are used extensively in baseball.

Proper first-aid and treatment procedures should be in writing, and there should be adequate provision for temporary care in case of injury or accident. All athletic contests should have competent trainers and, if possible, physicians in attendance.

Do Not Create Additional Hazards. Good leadership, adequate supervision, and common sense will reduce the chances of creating additional hazards. Proper crowd control through good precontest planning will also reduce the creation of hazards. Coaches today are better trained than in the past, but poor instruction in the fundamentals of a given activity is definitely a method of creating a hazard. Again it should be emphasized that when teaching any activity one should use a positive approach and first say, "This is the safe way to do this." The good coach, teacher, or sports administrator will use any measures that seem necessary for injury control in a specific situation.

Too many athletes have had a career ended or a season lost through injuries that might have been prevented if the hazards had been recognized, compensated for, or controlled.

football

Thousands of high schools in this country organize football teams, with over a million participating players. The very nature of the sport produces many injuries. Football is a game of vigorous exercise with lots of hard body contact. Many of the collisions are under high speed conditions.

Proper conditioning is a must in preventing football injuries. Most high school athletic associations prescribe a preseason conditioning program before allowing physical contact drills between players.

Coaches and athletic directors should buy only the best equipment for these young players. Although much protective equipment is available, it should be carefully selected and properly fitted.

Good leadership controls are needed. Most coaches feel that proper conditioning coupled with good equipment are the keys to holding accidents and injuries to a minimum.

Many types of surfaces are available for football fields. More research is needed to determine the effects on players of the different surfaces, and the types of equipment, especially shoes and headgear, that work best on each surface. Special care should be given to the selection of shoes and cleats.

Carl Blythe recommends the following for reducing and eliminating football injuries:

1. Mandatory medical examinations and medical history should be taken at the beginning of each season before allowing an athlete to participate in any football activity.
2. All personnel concerned with training football athletes should emphasize gradual and complete physical conditioning.
3. A physician should be present at all games and practice sessions. If it is impossible for a physician to be present at all practice sessions, emergency measures must be provided.
4. All personnel associated with football participation should be aware of the problems and safety measures related to physical activity in hot weather.
5. There should be continued emphasis on the employment of well trained athletic personnel and the provision of excellent facilities and the safest equipment possible.
6. There should be strict enforcement of game rules and administrative regulations in order to protect the health of the athlete. Coaches and school officials must support the game officials in their conduct of football activities.
7. Finally, there should be continued research concerning the safety factor in football.[37]

baseball and softball

Many serious and minor injuries occur each year in baseball, especially among younger players. (Very few deaths resulting directly from baseball have been reported.) One survey showed that approximately 82.5 percent of the injuries were of five different types: sprains, 27.3 percent; strains, 18.7 percent; contusions, 16.9 percent; pulled muscles, 11.3 percent; and fractures, 8.3 percent.[38]

Sliding and running between bases are the primary causes of sprains. Throwing and running between bases are common causes of strains. Contusions result mainly from being hit by a pitched ball, followed closely by collisions between players. Running between bases and throwing baseballs also produce many pulled muscles. Fractures are caused equally by sliding and by batters being hit by pitched balls.[39]

Ordinary participation in baseball and softball does not condition the player to the full extent necessary. Special exercises and much running are needed for proper physical conditioning. Many injuries could be reduced through conditioning programs.

[37] Carl Blythe, "Tackle Football," in *Sports Safety*, ed. C. P. Yost (Washington, D. C.: American Association for Health, Physical Education and Recreation, 1971), p. 96.

[38] Ronald G. Polk, "The Frequency and Causes of Baseball Injuries," *The Athletic Journal*, November 1968, pp. 19–20.

[39] Polk, "Baseball Injuries," p. 53.

Many baseball injuries could be eliminated by proper training in fundamentals. Sliding and base running present special problems. Protective equipment such as batting helmets should be used. With proper teaching and good leadership, baseball and softball can be played very safely with a minimum number of injuries.

basketball

Basketball players are vulnerable to injuries because basketball is a contact sport played under high speed conditions with very little protective equipment. In today's game, body contact under the baskets is often hard, and it comes at a time when players are off balance or in the air and therefore often not in the best positions to protect themselves.

Proper physical conditioning will reduce many injuries. Because of the length of the game and the conditions under which it is played, fatigue often becomes a big factor in causing injury.

Injuries come in many forms, but are not usually very serious. Death from a basketball accident is highly unusual. Sprains, strains, contusions, abrasions, and fractures are quite common. Adequate first aid and emergency care should be provided, with emphasis on control

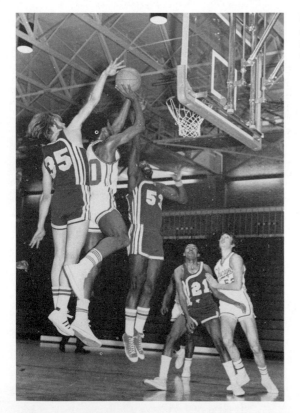

Figure 10-8. The play under the baskets is the roughest aspect of basketball. Photo courtesy of Chicago State University.

of infection. Infections resulting from injuries is apparently one of the big problems in basketball. Highly infectious abrasions usually occur when the player falls to a floor that contains dust or dirt from the shoes of other players.

Ample space should be provided all around the floor to keep players from colliding with walls or bleachers.

Basketball requires speed, agility, strength, and a combination of many skills. The fact that players are often required to rotate playing positions adds to the injury potential. Figure 10-8 depicts the action under the baskets in a game.

ice hockey

Ice hockey is said to be faster than basketball and rougher than football. Very few statistics are available on injuries related to the game. Players do reach very high speeds while skating, and often the contact is extremely hard. Players also suffer injuries from being hit by hockey sticks or pucks. Tempers frequently explode in this game, and fists often cause an injury.

Ice hockey is most popular in Canada and the northern United States. The construction of indoor ice-skating rinks in various parts of the country is making facilities available to more and more schools.

In recent years the number of high schools and colleges with ice hockey teams has increased. We can expect these increases to continue, especially since television has done much to popularize the sport. In larger cities there are many leagues now in operation. Not all the players are in good physical condition or have good equipment.

A reliable accident reporting system would help to make valid recommendations concerning the best ways to reduce injuries. Ice hockey injuries cover a wide range, including sprains, strains, contusions, fractures, and even deaths. Obviously both conditioning and the use of protective equipment are important. The equipment used in this sport is bulky and somewhat uncomfortable. The use of headgear is imperative. Many of the deaths from this sport could have been prevented had proper gear been worn.

track and field

Track and field is perhaps the safest of all team sports. Eighty percent of its injuries involve the legs, arms, feet, and hands.[40] The most

---

[40] Don C. Seaton, "Track and Field," in *Sports Safety*, ed. C. P. Yost (Washington, D. C.: American Association for Health, Physical Education and Recreation, 1971), p. 134.

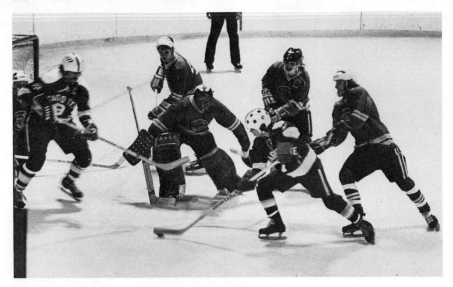

Figure 10-9. A hockey game in progress. Note the protective equipment worn by the players. Photo courtesy of Chicago State University.

dangerous events are the field events such as throwing the hammer, discus, and javelin.[41] High jumping and pole vaulting can be dangerous if the landing pits are not of good quality. The use of fiberglass poles has greatly increased the heights attainable by pole vaulting.

Proper conditioning and proper maintenance of the track and equipment are essential.

other sports

The reader should refer to Chapter 8 for a discussion of safety in individual sports, such as golf, tennis, swimming, and fishing.

SUMMARY

Although statistics regarding accidents to children while under school jurisdiction are insufficient, the data we do have indicates that the problem is serious. Our nation's schools must create safe school environments.

The failure to keep adequate accident records is a glaring weakness in our school safety programs. Accident record systems must be upgraded

[41] Seaton, "Track and Field," p. 134.

with provisions for a centralized system of collection and interpretation.

The fact that many, if not most, of our schools are not fire safe is a national disgrace. Schools are not functioning up to their potential in safety and safety education. By setting a good example of safety awareness in the school environment, schools can do much to make the individual safety conscious in later life.

Good master planning prior to construction of new facilities can greatly enhance our safety efforts in the future. School construction standards must be high. We cannot forsake safety for economy.

SUGGESTED STUDENT ACTIVITIES

1. Make a hazard analysis of selected areas around your school.
2. Make a task analysis of a skill such as defensive rebounding in basketball.
3. Study the records of evacuation times required in your school for possible remedial measures.
4. Design a playground with proper segregation of activities.
5. Find a hazard in your home or school and construct or provide adequate safeguards.
6. Study the accident records in your school and pinpoint the hazardous locations that need correcting.
7. Develop a to-and-from school route system.
8. Invite the supervisor of a school patrol system to speak to your class.
9. Analyze a parking lot to see if it meets state and federal standards.
10. Write a paper on safety in a selected sport. Develop your own principles of safety.

BIBLIOGRAPHY

AMERICAN ASSOCIATION FOR HEALTH, PHYSICAL EDUCATION AND RECREATION. *School Safety Policies with Emphasis on Physical Education, Athletics and Recreation.* Washington, D. C., 1968.

AMERICAN AUTOMOBILE ASSOCIATION. *How to Organize a School Safety Patrol.* Washington, D. C., 1960.

AMERICAN INSURANCE ASSOCIATION. *Safe Schools.* New York, 1968.

AUTOMOTIVE SAFETY FOUNDATION. *Guide to School Pedestrian Safety Program.* Washington, D. C., 1965.

BABCOCK, CHESTER I., and WILSON, REXFORD. *The Chicago School Fire.* Boston: National Fire Protection Association, 1959.

BLYTHE, CARL. "Tackle Football." In *Sports Safety,* edited by C. P. YOST.

Washington, D. C.: American Association for Health, Physical Education and Recreation, 1971.

CHICAGO MOTOR CLUB, TRAFFIC ENGINEERING DEPT. *School Safety Patrol Supervisors Manual.* Chicago, n.d.

CROSBY, R. W. and BLOCK, V. "How Safe Is the Ride to School?" *Traffic Safety,* October 1968, p. 13.

ENGELHARDT, NICKOLAUS L. *Complete Guide for Planning New Schools.* West Nyack, N. Y.: Parker Publishing Company, Inc., 1970.

MITTELSTAEDT, ARTHUR H., JR. "Planning School Grounds." *Journal of Health, Physical Education and Recreation* 40, No. 5 (May 1969), p. 37.

NATIONAL FIRE PROTECTION ASSOCIATION. *Occupancy Fire Record.* Fire Record FR 57-1A. Boston, 1965.

NATIONAL SAFETY COUNCIL. *Accident Facts 1973 Edition.* Chicago, 1973.

——. *Play Areas.* Safety Education Data Sheet No. 29. Chicago, n.d.

——. *School Bus Passengers Safety.* Safety Education Data Sheet No. 63. Chicago, n.d.

——. *School Emergency Procedures for Emergencies of Man Made Origin.* Safety Education Data Sheet No. 36. Chicago, n.d.

——. *School Fire Safety.* Safety Education Data Sheet No. 47 rev. Chicago, n.d.

——. *School Transportation: A Guide for Supervisors.* Chicago, 1967.

POLK, RONALD G. "The Frequency and Causes of Baseball Injuries." *The Athletic Journal,* November 1968, pp. 19–20, 53.

SEATON, DON C. "Track and Field." In *Sports Safety,* edited by C. P. YOST. Washington, D. C.: American Association for Health, Physical Education and Recreation, 1971.

STEWART, PAUL T. "The School and Pupil Transportation." *Traffic Safety,* July 1969, p. 12.

11

legal responsibility for school safety

Educators are concerned about the increasing number of lawsuits being brought against schools and school personnel. The probability that a public school teacher will be involved in court litigation arising out of a school-related pupil injury is greater today than at any other time in our history.[1] Because of the number of suits being initiated, all teachers and school administrators should understand the implications of lawsuits. They should also understand how to prevent such suits from occurring, and should know the possible defenses in the event that they do arise.

Liability for our purposes means being bound by law to make pecuniary remuneration for damages resulting from a tortious act. It is fundamental to the American way of life that people be held responsible for their wrongful acts, or "torts." [2]

> A tort is a legal wrong which proximately causes injury to person or property. The same act may be a crime and a tort. For example, the physical assault of one by another may be the crime of assault and battery (a wrong against the state), a penalty for which may be imposed through a criminal prosecution, and a tort (a civil or private wrong against the victim), damages for which may be assessed through civil proceedings.[3]

[1] Dennis J. Kigin, *Teacher Liability in School Shop Accidents* (Ann Arbor: Prakken Publications, Inc., 1973), p. 1.

[2] William R. Hazard, *Education and the Law* (New York: The Free Press, 1971), p. 405.

[3] Hazard, *Education and the Law*, p. 405.

A tortious act may be the result of misfeasance, malfeasance, or nonfeasance resulting in a breach of duty owed to another. Tortious acts therefore can include acts of commission or acts of omission.

Misfeasance is the improper or illegal performance of a legal act. For example, in a state where corporal punishment is legal, a teacher is guilty of misfeasance if he causes injury in the process of administering punishment by using a forbidden weapon such as his fist.

Malfeasance is the performance of an illegal act. Administering corporal punishment to a student in a state where such punishment is forbidden is malfeasance. In such a case the teacher would be subject to suit regardless of whether an injury occurred or not.

Nonfeasance is failure to perform a legal act that one ought to do. An example would be a teacher's failure to instruct pupils adequately in the necessary precautions for safe performance of a certain task, such as a tumbling stunt in gymnastics or a somewhat dangerous experiment in a chemistry class. Failing to provide the required supervision for the safety of students, such as leaving a classroom unattended, is another example of nonfeasance.

In most suits the teacher or school district will be charged with negligence, in which case it will be up to the plaintiff (the party making the charge) to prove that there was negligence and that it resulted in harm or injury. The law of negligence varies considerably from state to state.

SCHOOL LIABILITY

For years local government bodies, of which the school is an agent, have been free from tort liability under the doctrine of sovereign immunity. This archaic doctrine that the "king can do no wrong" originated in Europe and later found its way into American law. It denies the individual redress for any torts inflicted by the state or its instruments.[4] It is slowly disappearing from the American scene, however.

The advocates of government immunity argue that the school is an involuntary agent of local government, performing a service for the state that it is required to do by law. They also claim that since the school district operates on a nonprofit basis as an agent for the state and for the good of the state, the school district should enjoy the same immunity from suit without consent as does the sovereign state. Not only does the school operate from tax monies on a nonprofit basis, it is also forbidden to purchase insurance to protect itself against loss from negligence suits,

---

[4] Hazard, *Education and the Law*, p. 408.

on the theory that it would be improper for the school to spend tax appropriations for protection against something from which it is already immune by law.

An argument against sovereign immunity is that it is in conflict with our fundamental belief in "government by the consent of the governed." [5] Proponents of this position reason that the child is required by law to attend school, yet neither the child nor the parents have any control over the conditions at the school and therefore cannot protect themselves from injury.

Although there are many more arguments for and against this ancient doctrine, most authorities now believe that sovereign immunity is indefensible. Kenneth F. Licht said that any analogy between a king of England in 1765 and an American school district in 1970 is tenuous at best. [6]

Some states have either wholly or partially abrogated the doctrine of sovereign immunity. Abrogation usually begins with a court decision; formal approval is given later through legislative action. In many cases of partial abrogation the state legislatures arbitrarily set statutory limits on the amounts of the liability. The schools, in turn, purchase insurance to cover the maximum amount of liability permitted.

The wide variety in the methods of disposing of these suits makes it advisable for all educators to seek advice from their school attorneys to determine the relevant law in their particular state.

Despite the seemingly wide disagreement concerning liability, the most effective and cheapest protection is prevention. Without question, the threat of lawsuits has helped to upgrade school safety programs. In this limited way, the threat of lawsuits is commendable. However, this does not diminish the ethical responsibility for school safety programs.

TEACHER LIABILITY

The doctrine of sovereign immunity also directly affects the teacher. Under this doctrine school districts are not responsible for the acts of their employees. Industry, by way of contrast, is responsible for the acts of its employees under the doctrine of "respondeat superior." Some states that have abrogated the doctrine of sovereign immunity for schools have accepted liability for the negligence of their employees, in which case the school districts purchase insurance protection.

[5] Hazard, *Education and the Law*, p. 408.
[6] Kenneth F. Licht, "School Liability and Safety Education," *The Education Digest*, November 1970, p. 22.

In all states, however, the teachers themselves are subject to negligence suits, and in those states where the philosophy of respondeat superior does not apply, they stand alone in their defense. These cases are often tried by jury. Since juries are lay people with different backgrounds, their decisions vary from case to case even when the circumstances seem to be similar, and thus it is impossible to predict with accuracy what the outcome of a given suit may be.

NEGLIGENCE

The legal basis, and hence the success, of a negligence suit against a teacher rests on the plaintiff's ability to prove the charge. Negligence is defined as:

> the omission to do something which a reasonable man, guided by those considerations which ordinarily regulate human affairs, would do or the doing of something which a reasonable and prudent man would not do.[7]

In other words, did the teacher or defendant act as a reasonable and prudent person would have acted under those circumstances?

One element of negligence is foreseeability. Could the teacher have reasonably been expected to foresee that an accident resulting in pupil injury might happen? Did the teacher exercise reasonable and prudent care?

Teachers do have special privileges under the doctrine of "in loco parentis." As teachers, they can exercise parental authority over a child, in the absence of the parents, while the child is under school jurisdiction. However, they must take the same reasonable care to avoid an accident that a reasonable and prudent parent would take.

For example, a teacher may be obligated to stop a child from performing a dangerous act, such as swinging from a trapeze without proper protection, whereas an ordinary citizen witnessing the same event would have no authority to stop the act and could not be sued for failing to do so even though the child was injured. The "in loco parentis" doctrine, by the same token, would allow a teacher to administer corporal punishment if state statutes approve, whereas an ordinary citizen would be prohibited from doing so.

The critical question in such cases is whether, in the ordinary exercise of prudence and foresight, the teacher should have anticipated

---

[7] M. Chester Nolte and John Phillip Linn, *School Law for Teachers* (Danville, Ill.: The Interstate Printers and Publishers, Inc., 1963), p. 245.

trouble. If the answer is yes, then the teacher is negligent. If he or she could have anticipated trouble and failed to take preventive action, the teacher is imprudent and therefore negligent.[8]

A teacher's liability for damages is not limited to physical damages resulting from negligent action, but extends to liability for the following:

1. For physical harm resulting from fright or shock or other similar or immediate emotional disturbances caused by the injury or the negligent conduct causing it.
2. For additional bodily harm resulting from acts done by a third person in rendering aid irrespective of whether such acts are done in a proper or negligent manner.
3. For any disease which is contracted because of lowered vitality resulting from the injury caused by his negligent conduct.
4. For harm sustained in a subsequent accident which would not have occurred had the pupil's bodily efficiency not been impaired by the original negligence.[9]

Furthermore, the teacher may be liable for injuries resulting from his or her conduct even if the prior physical condition of the pupil is unknown.[10]

DEFENSES AGAINST NEGLIGENCE

Negligence in each case will be determined by the particular circumstances surrounding the event. As we know, there is a wide range in the final outcomes of negligence suits despite their seeming similarity. Juries and judges alike frequently disagree in their decisions. Following are some examples of possible defenses against negligence suits.

proximate cause or legal causation

If the conduct of a teacher is a substantial factor in bringing about the injury in question, there is no rule that relieves the liability. In other words the teacher's negligence is the legal cause of the injury.[11] However, to prove legal cause there must be an unbroken connection between the wrongful act and the injury. The sequence must be such as to make it

---

[8] Harry N. Rosenfield, *Guilty,* Special publication (Chicago: National Safety Council, 1963), p. 2.

[9] National Education Association, *Who Is Liable for Pupil Injuries?* (Washington, D. C., 1963), p. 15.

[10] National Education Association, *Who Is Liable?* p. 15.

[11] National Education Association, *Who Is Liable?* p. 11.

"just" to hold the teacher responsible for the injury suffered by the pupil.[12]

An example of this is a case where a student was fatally hurt, in the absence of a teacher, after he bumped heads with another player while jumping for a basketball. The court failed to find a causal connection between the absence of the teacher and the injury. It reasoned that the head bumping was a natural and normal possible consequence of the game that could not have been prevented had the teacher been present and given proper supervision.[13]

assumption of risk

The assumption of risk doctrine applies in those situations where a person, knowing the danger involved, voluntarily chooses to enter and remain within the area of risk.[14] Although courts do not often permit this defense, the following is an example of where the assumption of risk was held appropriate.

A high school freshman in a compulsory physical education class fell and broke his arm while playing leapfrog over a gymnasium horse. The teacher had instructed all the pupils on how to use the horse; had demonstrated the jump; had warned them of possible dangers; and had suggested that they not try the jump if they did not think they could safely do it. The teacher was held not liable since the pupil knew of the danger and voluntarily assumed the risk.[15]

This case illustrates the importance of giving adequate safety instruction to students when teaching any new technique or motor skill. Once again, precede all instruction in motor skills by saying "This is the safe way to do this," and then demonstrate. Such an approach would reduce the number of judgments for negligence against teachers.

contributory negligence

Did the injured party, through some misconduct of his own, contribute to the cause of the injury? If a pupil failed to take the precautions customarily expected of a person that age, the teacher cannot be held liable. In these cases the age of the pupil and the ability of a person that age to understand the inherent dangers may be the determining factors in deciding the issue.

[12] National Education Association, *Who Is Liable?* p. 11.
[13] National Education Association, *Who Is Liable?* pp. 11–12.
[14] National Education Association, *Who Is Liable?* p. 14.
[15] National Education Association, *Who Is Liable?* p. 15.

Contributory negligence is often invoked in pupil injury cases when the injury occurs on a street or highway after a pupil leaves the school bus. If a child of that particular age and experience should be capable of taking care of himself while crossing the street, most courts hold that his own negligence contributed to the injury.[16]

Some states have adopted a doctrine called "comparative negligence," which means that if the teacher's negligence is greater than that of the pupil the damages will be pro-rated. Again it should be pointed out that in either contributory negligence or comparative negligence, the age of the child will figure prominently in the ultimate decision.[17]

last clear chance

The "last clear chance" doctrine simply means that if the pupil had the final opportunity to prevent the accident and failed to do so, the teacher cannot be held liable. For example, if a pupil, through his own lack of concern, fails to stop while running in a gymnasium and consequently hits a wall, causing injury to himself, he may not be able to hold the teacher liable because he, and he alone, had the last clear chance to avoid the injury.

The test of foreseeability is a primary defense against negligence. In fact, the test of foreseeability *is* the test of negligence.

INSURANCE PROTECTION

The purpose of insurance is to protect against financial ruin. Today the insurance industry offers a variety of policies designed to that end. We are concerned with protection from liability arising out of a school-related pupil injury. The wide divergence in state laws and the increasing probability of a lawsuit make it advisable that teachers and other school personnel evaluate their particular situation to determine whether or not insurance protection is indicated. In those states where the doctrine of sovereign immunity has been abrogated, the school districts have accepted the responsibility for the acts of their employees; thus there is less need for the teacher to seek insurance protection.

The individual teacher is probably the most vulnerable to liability suits because of his or her unique position and constant contact with pupils. Liability insurance protection is available to the teacher in different forms. Some homeowner policies can be extended to offer broad

---

[16] National Education Association, *Who Is Liable?* p. 14.
[17] National Education Association, *Who Is Liable?* p. 14.

protection from all types of personal liability. Individual personal liability policies are also available at a very low cost, and many professional organizations offer them on a group basis to all members. Most importantly, the teacher should have adequate protection to cover any eventuality.

Many school districts subscribe to plans that allow parents to purchase insurance for their children on a group basis through the schools. The policies usually provide for medical expenses arising out of school-related injuries. The extent and type of coverage of these policies vary. They may prevent a lawsuit from arising, since provision is made to cover medical expenses, thereby eliminating the need to sue for that purpose.

Most schools today carry insurance to protect athletes and other special groups from financial loss due to injury. Driver education presents a special problem. All school districts should have ample coverage to provide complete financial protection in the event of an accident arising out of a driver education class. Driver education teachers should also check to see if any special insurance would be beneficial to them.

SUMMARY

In the final analysis the best defense against liability for negligence is prevention. Teachers should exercise extreme care and good judgment to prevent pupil injury. The very fact that they have made extensive efforts to prevent such injuries could in itself render them immune from liability. Filling out accident forms is important. Failure to do so is negligence in itself.

The threat of litigation arising from school-pupil-related injuries is a contributing force to the implementation of school safety programs. To that extent the threat of lawsuits is commendable. However, there are moral and ethical reasons why a school should make every effort to reduce pupil injuries.

As teachers' salaries go higher and as inflation continues to erode the dollar, the probability that a teacher will be brought into court as a result of a pupil injury will increase. Heightened public awareness and continued state abrogation of sovereign immunity will also give rise to these cases.

All educators and other school personnel should completely familiarize themselves with existing school liability codes in their particular states.

SUGGESTED STUDENT ACTIVITIES

1. Check the laws regarding sovereign immunity in your state and report back to your class.
2. Hold a mock trial in your class concerning a negligence suit.
3. Analyze the personal liability policies offered by at least three insurance companies, and compare their costs and benefits.
4. Check with the professional organizations in your area of specialization and determine what policies are available through them.
5. Write a paper on what insurance really does. Determine what is meant by "spreading of risk."
6. Review several court cases involving teachers in your area of specialization.

BIBLIOGRAPHY

HAZARD, WILLIAM R. *Education and the Law.* New York: The Free Press, 1971.

KIGIN, DENNIS J. *Teacher Liability in School Shop Accidents.* Ann Arbor: Prakken Publications, Inc., 1973.

LICHT, KENNETH F. "School Liability and Safety Education." Condensed from a release by the National Safety Council in *The Education Digest,* November 1970, p. 22.

NATIONAL EDUCATION ASSOCIATION. *Who Is Liable for Pupil Injuries?* Washington, D. C., 1963.

NOLTE, M. CHESTER, and LINN, JOHN PHILLIP. *School Law for Teachers.* Danville, Ill.: The Interstate Printers and Publishers, Inc., 1963.

ROSENFIELD, HARRY N. *Guilty.* Special publication. Chicago: National Safety Council, 1963.

12

disaster readiness

Disasters occur in unpredictable fashion, usually without warning, often causing heavy loss of life and destruction of property. Some disasters are blamed on the forces of nature; others are caused by man himself. Regardless of the source, the enormity of devastation caused by disasters makes it imperative that we plan in order to reduce these effects and to promote faster and more efficient recovery.

Over the years there have been more than 100 pieces of federal legislation, mostly remedial in nature, dealing with disasters. Since about 1950, as a result of past experience and research and the ever-present possibility of enemy attack, planning for disasters has become more sophisticated. In a form of government such as in the United States, effective planning should originate at the federal level; however, all levels of government must cooperate closely.

To meet the threat of enemy attack, Congress in 1950 established an independent federal agency known as the Federal Civil Defense Administration. This agency was designed to stimulate and assist states and local communities in making plans to minimize the effects of disaster and to advance the training of volunteer personnel. During the next eleven years the civil defense program was reorganized several times, adding to its scope and clarity. In 1961, by executive order of the president, civil defense activities were transferred to the Department of Defense and administered by its Office of Civil Defense. This gave official recognition to civil defense as an integral part of the total defense effort. In 1964 the secretary of defense transferred the Office of Civil Defense to the Office of the Secretary of the Army.[1]

Today there is also an Office of Emergency Preparedness in the executive office of the president. It deals primarily with natural disasters, but maintains close liaison with the Office of Civil Defense.

NATURAL DISASTERS

Natural disasters come in many forms—tornadoes, cyclones, earthquakes, floods, hurricanes, blizzards, and others. Table 12-1 lists the major disasters that have affected the United States in previous years.

Preparing for natural disasters begins with recognizing and understanding what types are likely to occur in a given area.[2] Based on this premise, the first step in adequate emergency preparedness for any community would be an analysis of vulnerability. Some areas of the country are subject to hurricanes; others experience tornadoes; still others are struck by earthquakes, volcanic eruptions, floods, forest fires, or blizzards.

Although an individual disaster is impossible to predict, the types of disasters most likely to occur in an area can be predetermined with some accuracy. For example, Florida can reasonably expect hurricanes, while New England can expect blizzards. Some areas of the country, such as the Midwest, are susceptible to many different types of natural disasters. Vulnerability analysis is an essential step in the planning for disaster preparedness.[3]

An analysis of vulnerability should include the possibilities of man-made disasters, such as fire or explosions. An area containing oil refineries or chemical plants, for instance, should make extensive preparations for fire and explosion. Nuclear reactor plants present special problems. Many communities (mining towns, for example) contain some type of business that has a potential for disaster.

One of the weaknesses in disaster planning on a state and national basis has been the lack of systematic vulnerability analysis. As a result, many communities are not as well prepared as they should be.[4] Another weakness is that most communities tend to rely on civil defense organizations for total community planning. In certain cases this may be satisfactory, but it should be recognized that civil defense plans are primarily

[1] National School Boards Association, *School Boards Plan for Civil Defense* (Evanston, Ill., 1965), p. 6.
[2] Office of Emergency Preparedness, *Disaster Preparedness: Report to Congress* (Washington, D. C., 1972), 1:9.
[3] Office of Emergency Preparedness, *Disaster Preparedness,* 1:9.
[4] Office of Emergency Preparedness, *Disaster Preparedness,* 1:9.

Table 12-1. Major disasters in previous years.

Type and Location	No. of Deaths	Date of Disaster
Fires:		
Peshtigo, Wisc. and surrounding area forest fire	1,152	Oct. 9, 1871
Iroquois Theatre, Chicago	575	Dec. 30, 1903
Boston night club	492	Nov. 28, 1942
North German Lloyd Steamships, Hoboken, N.J.	326	June 30, 1900
Ohio penitentiary, Columbus	320	Apr. 21, 1930
Cloquet, Minn. and surrounding area forest fire	283	Oct. 12, 1918
City of Chicago	250	Oct. 9, 1871
Dance hall, Natchez, Mississippi	208	Apr. 23, 1940
Hartford, Conn. circus	168	July 6, 1944
Atlanta hotel	119	Dec. 7, 1946
Marine:		
"Sultana" exploded—Mississippi River	1,547	Apr. 27, 1865
"Titanic" struck iceberg—Atlantic Ocean	1,517	Apr. 15, 1912
"Empress of Ireland" ship collision—St. Lawrence River	1,024	May 29, 1914
"General Slocum" burned—East River	1,021	June 15, 1904
"Eastland" capsized—Chicago River	812	July 24, 1915
"Morro-Castle" burned—off New Jersey coast	134	Sept. 8, 1934
U. S. Carrier "Bennington" exploded—off Rhode Island coast	103	May 26, 1954
Floods:		
Galveston tidal wave	6,000	Sept. 8, 1900
Johnstown, Pa.	2,209	May 31, 1889
Ohio and Indiana	732	Mar. 28, 1913
St. Francis, Calif. dam burst	450	Mar. 13, 1928
Ohio and Mississippi River valleys	360	Jan. 22, 1937
Texas	215	Sept. 6-10, 1921
Los Angeles	181	Mar. 2, 1938
Ohio, Allegheny, Monongahela and Susquehanna Rivers	168	Mar. 18-24, 1936
Rapid City, S. Dak. flash flood	237	June 9, 1972
Storms:		
Florida hurricane	1,833	Sept. 16-17, 1928
New England hurricane	657	Sept. 21, 1938
Illinois tornado	606	Mar. 18, 1925
Louisiana hurricane	500	Sept. 29, 1915
Florida hurricane	409	Sept. 1-2, 1935
Miss., Ala. and Ga. tornadoes	402	Apr. 2-7, 1936
Louisiana and Texas hurricane	395	June 27-28, 1957
Texas coast hurricane	375	Aug. 16, 1915
Texas hurricane	287	Sept. 14-17, 1919
Ind., Ohio, Mich., Ill. and Wisc. tornadoes	272	Apr. 11, 1965
Gulf coast (Fla., Ala., Miss.) hurricane	243	Sept. 17-18, 1926
Ark., Tenn., Mo., Miss., and Ala. tornadoes	229	Mar. 21-22, 1952
Mississippi and Louisiana hurricane	200	Aug. 17, 1969
Northeastern states hurricane	180	Aug. 17-19, 1955
Texas-Oklahoma tornado	167	Apr. 9, 1947
Pa., W.Va. and Md. tornadoes	159	June 23, 1944
Mississippi and Louisiana tornadoes	117	Feb. 21, 1971
Others:		
Texas City, Texas ship explosion	561	Apr. 16, 1947
San Francisco earthquake and fire	452	Apr. 18, 1906
Port Chicago, Calif. ship explosion	322	July 18, 1944
New London, Texas school explosion	294	Mar. 18, 1937
Two-plane collision over New York City	134	Dec. 16, 1960
Cleveland gas tank explosion	130	Oct. 20, 1944
Two-plane collision over Grand Canyon, Arizona	128	June 30, 1956
Long Beach, Calif. earthquake	120	Mar. 10, 1933
Alaska earthquake	117	Mar. 27, 1964
Scheduled jetliner crash into mountainside near Juneau, Alaska	111	Sept. 4, 1971

Source: National Almanac, World Almanac, National Fire Protection Assn., Chicago Historical Society, Texas Inspection Bureau, American Red Cross, city and state Boards of Health, and the Metropolitan Life Insurance Company.

Reproduced from Accident Facts 1973 Edition, *p. 21, courtesy of the National Safety Council.*

for protection and recovery in the event of nuclear attack. They are usually developed on the basis that there will be little if any help from the outside, due to the probable general immobility of the entire community caused by severe blast damage and radioactive fallout over the entire area. But in planning for natural disasters, the opposite assumption can be made. Help from the outside will be a likely possibility. There will be movement and evacuation and a place to go.[5]

Food supply is a good example of the difference between planning for a natural disaster and planning for a nuclear attack. Food supplies should be stocked in shelters constructed for use in the event of nuclear attack. In the case of natural disaster, emergency food supplies should be kept out of the area of the potential disaster since they can be readily moved in later, thereby reducing the possibility of contamination.

Many federal agencies can give communities assistance in vulnerability analysis. For example, the Army Corps of Engineers provides valuable assistance in flood prevention and preparedness; the National Oceanic and Atmospheric Administration (NOAA) conducts vulnerability surveys of coastal communities with a high risk of hurricanes.[6]

Once the vulnerability analysis is completed, emergency procedures should be set up to reduce loss of life, injury, and property damage. Plans for emergency responses to major disasters should focus on:

1. Expansion of routine emergency services, such as police, fire fighting, and sanitation.
2. Provisions for items that individual citizens themselves take care of under normal conditions, such as food, housing, clothing, and personal welfare.
3. Special provisions for medical care.[7]

Obviously, planning for these emergencies involves many government agencies as well as private groups. A well-planned emergency response system enhances the proper execution of control and recovery procedures under emergency conditions. Poor planning results in panic, chaos, needless injuries and loss of life, and increased property damage. The importance of a well-planned emergency procedure cannot be overemphasized. There is ample evidence that planning for emergencies does pay off.

Past experience has taught many things about disasters, and all available scientific and technological knowledge should be applied. Research is currently being carried on concerning the characteristics of different types of disasters. It is now the general practice to rush research personnel to the scene of a disaster to collect data that might help to reduce loss of life and property damage in similar future disasters. This

[5] Office of Emergency Preparedness, *Disaster Preparedness*, 1:9.
[6] Office of Emergency Preparedness, *Disaster Preparedness*, 1:9.
[7] Office of Emergency Preparedness, *Disaster Preparedness*, 1:5.

data must, of course, be gathered prior to cleanup operations. Undoubtedly such research will provide many answers, especially in the area of building construction and prevention and recovery procedures.

Radar is proving invaluable in detecting certain weather phenomena, such as tornadoes and movements of air masses. Space programs and other research may add much knowledge to weather forecasting and possibly even weather modification. It may one day be possible to change the direction of a hurricane, for example, and route the storm away from highly populated cities to an area of drought. Reducing the intensity of wind could lessen property damage. Reducing the amount of lightning could reduce fires. Weather modification is a new and exciting area with unlimited possibilities and unforeseen consequences.[8]

Each disaster has individual characteristics that make planning for it unique. However, there are certain specific postdisaster recommendations that can be applied, regardless of the type of natural disaster. Some precautions for natural disaster situations are:

1. Use extreme caution in entering or working in buildings that may have been structurally weakened.
2. Be careful with matches, lanterns, torches, and lighted cigarettes because of the possibility of gas leaks, or the presence of flammable material.
3. Check for leaking gas in your home. Do this by smell only.
4. Stay away from fallen or damaged electric wires, since they may be dangerous.
5. If you have electrical appliances that are wet, turn off the main power switch and then unplug the appliances.
6. Check all food and water supplies before using them. Food in refrigerators may have spoiled while the electricity was off. Do not eat any food that has been in contact with flood water.
7. If needed, get food, water, clothing, and medical care at a Red Cross station or from local government authorities.
8. Stay away from disaster areas. Sightseeing can be dangerous and can interfere with rescue operations.
9. Don't drive unless necessary. Report any driving hazards to local authorities.
10. Do not pass rumors or exaggerated reports of damage.
11. Follow the advice and instructions of your local government.[9]

[8] Office of Emergency Preparedness, *Disaster Preparedness*, 1:6.
[9] Department of Defense, Office of Civil Defense, *In Time of Emergency* (Washington, D. C., 1968), pp. 73–74.

tornadoes

Tornadoes are local atmospheric storms, generally short in duration, formed by winds rotating at very high speeds, usually in a counterclockwise direction. These storms may appear as a vortex or whirlpool-like column of winds rotating about a hollow cavity in which centrifugal forces produce a partial vacuum.

The tornado occurs with severe thunderstorms. Tornado funnels appear as extensions of the dark, heavy cumulonimbus thunderstorm clouds, and the funnels extend downward to the ground.[10] Technically the funnel must touch the ground to be called a tornado. The same condition appearing over water is called a waterspout.

Usually tornado paths are only about an eighth of a mile wide and seldom more than 10 miles long.[11] However, tornadoes have caused heavy destruction along paths of over a mile wide and upward of 300 miles long. One tornado traveled 293 miles across the states of Illinois and Indiana on May 26, 1917. It lasted seven hours and twenty minutes. Its forward speed was 40 miles an hour, an average figure for tornadoes.[12]

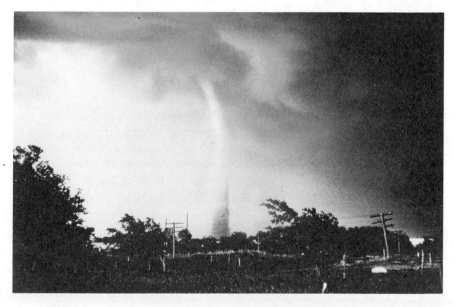

Figure 12-1. *A tornado funnel cloud. Photo courtesy of the U.S. Department of Commerce, National Oceanic and Atmospheric Administration.*

[10] Office of Emergency Preparedness, *Disaster Preparedness*, 3:27.
[11] Office of Emergency Preparedness, *Disaster Preparedness*, 3:28.
[12] Office of Emergency Preparedness, *Disaster Preparedness*, 3:28.

Most authorities agree that tornadoes are the most violent and destructive weather phenomena known to man. Their high wind velocity and pressure differentials make them especially hazardous. Since they strike with suddenness, the advance warning period is short.

A tornado needs special atmospheric conditions in order to form. There must be layers of air with contrasting characteristics of temperature, density, moisture, and wind flow. Several theories have been advanced about the type of energy transformation necessary to create a tornado. The two most frequently quoted theories credit tornado formation to either the effect of thermally induced rotary circulations or the mechanical effect of converging rotary winds. Most scientists seem to feel that a combination of thermal and mechanical effects generates a tornado.[13]

Tornadoes seem to follow a pattern. The months of greatest frequency are April, May, and June. In February, when tornado activity starts to increase, most of these storms occur in the central Gulf region. During March the area of maximum frequency moves eastward to the southeast Atlantic Coast states, where the occurrences peak in April. During May they move to the Southern Plains, and in June to the Northern Plains and Great Lakes area, and even as far east as the western part of New York. The reason for these shifts is said to be the increasing penetration of warm moist air masses from the south into the continental land mass, while contrasting cool air surges in from the north and northeast. Tornadoes tend to be generated most frequently during a collision of these air masses.[14]

Emergency information regarding tornadoes usually begins with a "watch," which is a forecast predicting the probability of these storms in a given area. A "warning" means that a tornado has actually been sighted; it gives the location, the area that could be affected, and the predicted duration of the tornado in the area. People should remain calm and seek shelter immediately in the event of a warning in their locale.

The following instructions should be followed if a tornado occurs:

1. Open windows and doors on the side of the structure *away* from the tornado. This will help to equalize pressure differentials against the walls and may save the building from collapsing.
2. If possible get underground, preferably in a basement, storm cellar, underground parking lot, or subway. If at home go to the corner of the basement *nearest* the tornado.

[13] Office of Emergency Preparedness, *Disaster Preparedness*, 3:27–28.
[14] Office of Emergency Preparedness, *Disaster Preparedness*, 3:31.

3. Schools and buildings may have shelters; if so use them. If not, go to interior hallways, in the basement if possible. Stay away from windows. Avoid gymnasiums, auditoriums, or other structures with wide, free span roofs.
4. Cars are dangerous. If you are traveling in a car in open country and time permits, you may be able to drive at right angles to the tornado and escape. It might be best, however, to leave the car and find a ground depression to lie in.

windstorms

Windstorms represent the same type of problems as tornadoes, and the same precautions apply.

hurricanes

Hurricanes are large revolving storms accompanied by violent destructive winds, heavy rains, and high waves and tides. They are known by different names in different parts of the world, such as typhoons or tropical cyclones, but they all belong to the same general family. These storms are common along the southern and eastern coast of the United States and in the Atlantic Ocean, the Caribbean Sea, and the Gulf of Mexico.

Hurricanes originate over water close to the equator, where there is warm and moist air. The first indication of a coming storm is usually a vast area of unsettled weather. The air begins to move toward and around a central area where barometric pressure is falling, gradually assuming a circular (counterclockwise in the northern hemisphere) motion around a center of lowest pressure. The mass begins to move somewhat like a top spinning across a smooth surface. The circular motion becomes more violent as the storm develops, often reaching speeds in excess of 100 miles an hour, with a forward motion of 10 to 15 miles an hour. The area of destruction along the path of the hurricane may be 25 to 500 miles wide. Usually, warning of a hurricane comes well in advance of its approach toward any area in this country. Once it is known that a hurricane is forming, the weather bureau begins to broadcast "advisories" day and night.

Safety measures to be followed in the event of a hurricane are:

1. Keep radio or television tuned in for weather advisories.
2. Keep on hand an ample supply of food that can be eaten without cooking. Canned foods are recommended.

3. Vacate low-lying beaches and do not enter areas subject to high tidal waves.
4. Make provisions for an ample supply of water, and be sure emergency cooking facilities are working.
5. If possible have emergency lighting facilities.
6. Keep a sufficient quantity of gasoline in your car, since service stations may be shut down for a long time after the storm.
7. Create an opening in the house on the opposite side from the storm.
8. Board up windows or use storm shutters.
9. Pay no attention to rumors. Remain calm and listen to official broadcasts.
10. Well-built homes away from the dangers of tidal waves are probably the best protection.[15]

blizzards

Blizzards are common to many of our northern states. They differ from ordinary snowstorms in that they are usually accompanied by high winds, fine snow, and extremely cold temperatures. This combination causes many deaths and injuries each year because people are unable to reach shelter in time. Although blizzards can form quickly, there is usually sufficient advance warning from weather forecasters. Most deaths could be prevented if proper precautions were taken. It is common in northern states for factories and offices to dismiss workers early in anticipation of a blizzard. People living in areas where blizzards are almost a yearly occurrence should keep at least a week's supply of food on hand during the winter months.

Some tips to follow in case you are caught in a car during a blizzard are:

1. Do not leave the car. State and county patrols with proper equipment begin immediate searches for marooned cars.
2. Run the motor occasionally to warm the car, but be sure to open a window for ventilation. If possible keep snow from piling up behind the car and preventing the exhaust system from functioning. If this happens you cannot run the car. Try to save on gasoline.
3. If the car runs out of gas, close all the windows immediately and stuff handkerchiefs or the like in all cracks.

[15] National Safety Council, *Safety in Bad Weather Conditions*, Safety Education Data Sheet No. 76 (Chicago, n.d.).

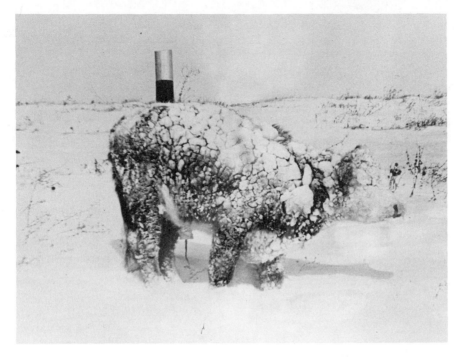

Figure 12-2. A blizzard condition. Photo courtesy of the U.S. Department of Commerce, National Oceanic and Atmospheric Administration.

4. Do not open car doors after you run out of gas, and under no circumstances go to sleep.
5. Exercise occasionally by stamping your feet.
6. Remove your shoes and massage your feet if they get too cold.
7. Most of all, remain calm until help arrives.

People living in blizzard areas should carry emergency kits in their cars with food rations, warm socks, heavy mittens, and other articles.[16]

floods

Many areas of the United States are subject to floods, especially the lowlands along the Mississippi and other major rivers. Much progress has been made in flood prevention through the use of dams and dikes. There is always advance warning of a flood, except in the case of flash floods. Proper action will practically eliminate loss of life and will cut down on property losses.

[16] National Safety Council, *Safety in Bad Weather Conditions.*

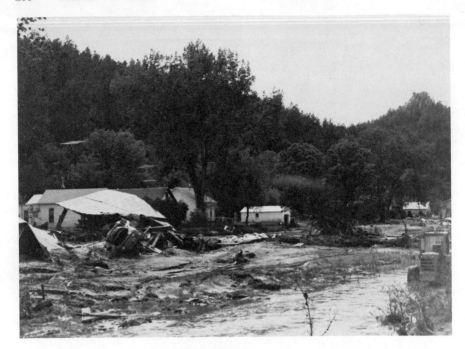

Figure 12-3. A flood condition. Photo courtesy of the U.S. Department of Commerce, National Oceanic and Atmospheric Administration.

If you live in areas where floods do occur, you should do the following:

1. Follow the instructions and advice of the local government.
2. Secure your home before leaving, and if you have time bring outside possessions inside the house or tie them down securely.
3. Board up windows.
4. Do not stack sandbags around the outside walls of the house. This can cause houses with basements to suffer severe damage or float off the foundation.
5. Travel with care.
6. Leave home early enough to avoid being marooned.
7. Make sure you have plenty of gas in your car.
8. Follow recommended routes.[17]

earthquakes

An earthquake can be one of nature's most devastating phenomena. Earthquakes releasing enough energy to cause readings of 8.5 on the

[17] Department of Defense, *In Time of Emergency*, pp. 75–77.

Richter scale are equivalent to 12,000 times the energy released by the Hiroshima nuclear bomb in 1945. Although the focus of a quake is well below the earth's surface, cities have been destroyed and thousands of lives lost in only a few seconds.[18]

The first warning of an earthquake is a deep rumbling or disturbed air making a rushing sound, followed by a series of violent motions in the ground. Often the ground fissures, and there can be large displacements —21 feet horizontally in San Francisco in 1906 and 47 feet vertically at Yakutat Bay, Alaska, in 1899.[19] Earthquakes can happen in several areas of the United States, but are more likely to occur in the Pacific region and some other western states. Scientists have constructed "risk maps" that show the areas of the country most likely to have earthquakes.

Much can be done to prevent death, injury, and damage from earthquakes through proper planning and use of the susceptible ground. Good building construction in possible earthquake areas would reduce property damage. Many cities in California have stringent building codes for suspect areas.

Although the shaking of the ground may be frightening during an earthquake, you have an excellent chance of survival if you take a few precautions. Here are some things to remember:

1. Remain calm. Do not run or panic.
2. Stay where you are. If you are outdoors, stay outdoors; if indoors, stay indoors. Most people get hurt entering or leaving buildings during earthquakes, usually from being hit with falling objects or electric wires.
3. If indoors, sit or stand against an inside wall, preferably in the basement, or take cover under a heavy piece of furniture, such as a desk, table, or bench.
4. If you are outdoors, stay away from overhead electric wires, poles, or anything that might fall.
5. If you are driving an automobile, pull off the road and stop.[20]

MAN-MADE DISASTERS

Man-made disasters include such things as riots, civil disturbances, fire (which is discussed in a separate chapter), and war. Wars are the most destructive of all man-made disasters, and the discovery of nuclear weapons has increased their destructive potential many fold.

[18] Office of Emergency Preparedness, *Disaster Preparedness*, 3:72.
[19] Office of Emergency Preparedness, *Disaster Preparedness*, 3:72.
[20] Department of Defense, *In Time of Emergency*, pp. 85–86.

riots and civil disturbances

Riots and civil disturbances have been taking place since the beginning of mankind. No area of the world is immune to this type of disaster. For the most part, they have not been as destructive as other forms of disasters; however, in recent years civil disturbances in various places in the world have taken on more serious consequences. They stem from man's inability to communicate and settle his differences on a rational basis.

Some things to remember for riot protection are:

1. Be alert to the social setting.
2. Guard against false rumors.
3. Avoid areas where riots are taking place. Let the police and other agencies handle the situation.
4. Go into seclusion, if necessary.

Schools should take these extra precautions:

1. Devise safe exit routes for students and employees.
2. Lock boiler rooms and power equipment when not in use.
3. Provide adequate lighting for the exterior and interior of the school.
4. Consider increasing the supply and availability of dry chemical fire extinguishers.
5. Locate duplicates of important papers in safe areas outside the school.
6. Keep flammable liquids and materials isolated and stored according to local fire codes.
7. Keep police and fire department phone numbers at the school switchboard.

nuclear attack

In the event of an enemy attack with nuclear weapons, the main effects would be intense light (flash), heat (which would start many fires), blast, and radiation. The intensity of these effects would depend on the size and type of explosion, the weather conditions, the terrain (whether the ground is flat or hilly), and the height of the explosion.[21]

People close to the explosion would be killed or very seriously

[21] Department of Defense, *In Time of Emergency*, p. 10.

injured by the blast or the heat of the nuclear fireball. To people in the fringe areas (a few miles away), blast, heat, and fires started by the explosion would be dangerous. However, most people in the fringe areas would probably survive.[22]

Outside the fringe areas, people would not be affected by the blast, heat, or fire, but would be subject to radioactive fallout. Department of Defense studies indicate that in any nuclear attack on this country, tens of millions of Americans would be outside the fringe areas.[23]

When nuclear weapons explode near the ground, great quantities of pulverized earth and debris are sucked up into the mushroom-type nuclear cloud. Radioactive gases produced by the explosion condense on and into the debris, producing radioactive fallout particles. These particles then fall back to the ground, giving off invisible gamma rays (like X rays). Overexposure to these rays can kill or injure people.[24]

Weather factors such as wind currents will determine the distribution pattern of fallout particles. Therefore, there is no way to predict how soon, or to what extent, the particles would fall back to earth at a given location. Any area in the United States might be subject to some fallout. Certain communities might get heavy accumulations, while others nearby might get very little. Areas close to the explosion might get fallout within 15 to 30 minutes, while it might take 5 to 10 hours for the particles to reach a community 100 to 200 miles away.[25]

Probably the first 24 hours would be the most dangerous from the standpoint of fallout. The heavier particles would tend to fall quickly and still be highly radioactive, thus giving off strong rays. The lighter particles, which stay airborne longer, would lose much of their radiation high in the atmosphere.[26]

Radioactive fallout is a manageable problem, providing that proper precautions are taken. Some fallout will be visible and some too fine to be seen. Fallout does damage living things, such as plants and animals, but it does not make them radioactive. You cannot catch "radiation sickness" from another person.[27]

Fallout gives off three types of radiation: alpha, beta, and gamma. All three can be blocked with sufficient shielding. For example, alpha radiation can be stopped by a sheet of paper, and beta radiation by ordinary clothing. Gamma radiation is the biggest problem and requires more dense shielding.[28] The federal government provides information concern-

[22] Department of Defense, *In Time of Emergency*, pp. 10–11.
[23] Department of Defense, *In Time of Emergency*, p. 11.
[24] Department of Defense, *In Time of Emergency*, p. 11.
[25] Department of Defense, *In Time of Emergency*, p. 12.
[26] Department of Defense, *In Time of Emergency*, p. 12.
[27] National School Boards Association, *Plan for Civil Defense*, p. 9.
[28] National School Boards Association, *Plan for Civil Defense*, pp. 9–10.

ing the proper types of materials to prevent overexposure to radioactive fallout.

Following is a checklist of emergency actions:

1. Know your local emergency action plan.
2. Understand nuclear attack and hazards.
3. Know the attack warning signal.
4. Know the location of fallout shelters.
5. If no shelter is available, improvise protection.
6. Prepare emergency supplies.
7. Conserve emergency supplies; maintain sanitation.
8. Reduce fire hazards.
9. Know the basics of emergency medical care.
10. Follow official instructions.[29]

CIVIL DEFENSE PLANNING

The purpose of civil defense is to develop plans for coordinated action that will give maximum protection to the population in periods of emergency. Civil defense calls for the utilization of the existing government structure adapted to meet emergency needs.[30] As noted before, it requires a different type of preparation from that required for natural disasters.

There would be no need for civil defense if man would act in a rational manner, but man does not always act or react in a rational manner, as evidenced by the number of wars over the years.[31]

Advanced technology gave man the ability to release nuclear energy. With this came an almost inexhaustible source of power and an array of nuclear weapons capable of great destruction. These weapons, if unleashed, can cause more destruction than any other form of man-made devastation. In reality there can be no complete security should these weapons be used. Great numbers of lives would certainly be lost. Therefore, man must devise methods of maximum protection in the event of nuclear attack.[32]

Effective civil defense requires advance planning at all levels of government—local, state, and national. The plans must be flexible enough to accommodate any changes in enemy tactics and weapons, and compre-

---

[29] Department of Defense, *In Time of Emergency*, pp. 6–7.
[30] National Education Association, *Schools and Civil Defense* (Washington, D. C., 1964), p. 8.
[31] National Education Association, *Schools and Civil Defense*, p. 8.
[32] National Education Association, *Schools and Civil Defense*, p. 8.

hensive enough to cover millions of people living under widely different conditions.

national planning

To facilitate civil defense planning, the federal government, through the Office of Civil Defense, has assumed four responsibilities, namely:

1. To keep track of the nature of the threat that civil defense programs must meet.
2. To prepare and disseminate information about the threat and how it can be met.
3. To bear a major part of the cost of certain kinds of civil defense activities.
4. To provide technical assistance through state and local channels for civil defense planning.[33]

One of the major elements in a civil defense plan is the establishment of a national system of fallout shelters. This responsibility lies with the Office of Civil Defense, along with postattack assistance, communications and alert systems, and others. Planning for radiological warfare defenses and the like must of necessity also be done at the national level.

state planning

State and local governments have the major operating responsibility for civil defense. State governors are responsible for these programs, and in most states there is a state director who coordinates the work within his state and works with authorities in surrounding states.

Some additional state responsibilities would be to:

1. Determine requirements of the state and its political subdivisions for food, clothing, and other needs.
2. Procure and pre-position supplies, medicines, machines, material, and equipment.
3. Promulgate standards and requirements for local and interjurisdictional disaster plans. Periodically review local plans.
4. Provide for mobile support units.
5. Assist with local training programs.
6. Make surveys of public and private industries, resources, and facilities.

[33] National Education Association, *Schools and Civil Defense*, p. 9.

7. Plan and make arrangements for the availability of public and private facilities.
8. Establish a register of persons with types of training and skill important in emergency prevention.
9. Establish a register of available mobile and construction equipment and temporary housing.
10. Do other things necessary for proper civil defense planning and execution.[34]

local planning

In the final analysis, the effectiveness of any civil defense plans will be determined by how well the plan is executed at the local level. Should the occasion arise, it will be the local civil defense organization that issues directives to the population concerning where to go and what to do. It will also be responsible, with state and national support, for the initiation of postattack procedures.

Effective execution of such a plan in case of emergency will require in-depth advance planning and training of personnel. The nation's schools will play a major role in the event of disaster; therefore they must work closely with local civil defense authorities. Schools are natural centers for emergency hospitals or fallout shelters. Moreover, it is possible that millions of children could be in the schools during an attack. Schools also carry a major responsibility for education for civil defense.

Every school should have plans that are in complete harmony with the over-all plans of the local community. The board of education has the responsibility for school planning and should begin with a statement of policy concerning civil defense, followed by the definite assignment of responsibility for planning and organization. School plans should provide for all possible eventualities.

The size of the school system will determine the type of school plan utilized. Figure 12-4 illustrates a suggested organization plan. It can be modified to fit the local situation.

warning and communications systems

In all probability, an attack on the United States by a foreign power would follow a period of international tension. This should serve to keep the citizenry alert to the possibility of attack. An attack would be detected by our network of warning systems in time to allow at least some people to get to fallout shelters. The warning could be very short, but it also

---

[34] Office of Emergency Preparedness, *Disaster Preparedness*, 2:12.

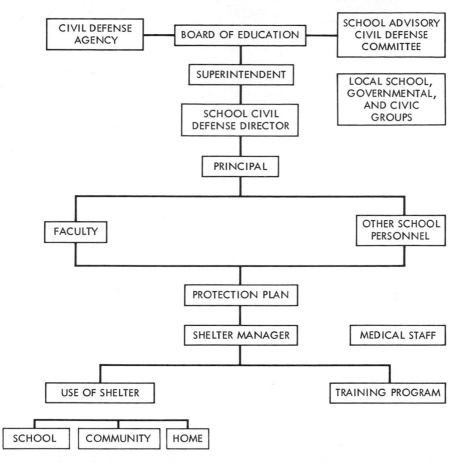

Figure 12-4. *An organization chart for school civil defense. From* School Boards Plan for Civil Defense, *courtesy of the National School Boards Association.*

could come well in advance of an attack. There are several different ways in which you might receive warnings of attack, including word of mouth. Many United States cities have warning systems using sirens, whistles, or horns. You should be familiar with the signals in your community, since they are often used to warn people of a natural disaster, such as a tornado.

ATTACK WARNING SIGNAL. This will be sounded only in event of enemy attack. The signal is a 3- to 5-minute wavering sound of the sirens or a series of short blasts on whistles or horns (see Figure 12-5). This means that an actual attack against the United States has been detected and that protective action should be taken at once.

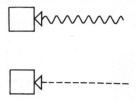

Figure 12-5. Attack warning signals.

EMERGENCY BROADCAST SYSTEMS. Selected radio stations have been licensed to make emergency broadcasts over standard frequencies in the event of nuclear attack. These stations will broadcast vital information to the public. They will not identify themselves by call letters, but will give their location. Since power failure is a distinct possibility during enemy attack, it is imperative that people keep transistor radios on hand and in good working condition. Every school, hospital, and other public institution should have transistor radios. They are a must for fallout shelters. People should listen to these broadcasts and refrain from using the telephone if at all possible.

SUMMARY

Disaster readiness is more important in our modern society than at any other time in history. Nuclear weapons with sophisticated delivery systems make any nation vulnerable to possible attack. The concentration of population in urban centers complicates the potential of natural disasters.

Proper planning for disasters represents our best opportunity to deal with these events. A well-organized plan promotes safe and efficient recovery. With today's advanced technology, increased medical knowledge, and vulnerability analysis, the possible effects of disaster can be greatly reduced. Every community must have such a plan.

Proper planning for disasters requires cooperation among national, state, and local communities. Every agency within the community should be involved. Good planning may prevent many man-made disasters. If your community does not have an adequate plan, try to initiate a program. The cost of planning is cheap compared to the possible good it can do.

SUGGESTED STUDENT ACTIVITIES

1. Make a list of the possible disasters that might logically occur in your community.

2. Check with local governmental officials and learn about their planning effort in your community.

3. Develop a disaster plan for your school.

4. If possible visit a disaster communications control center.

5. Plan a fallout shelter for your family and list all the needs.

6. Write a term paper on radioactive fallout and the effects of the different rays.

7. Invite a civil defense official to speak before your class.

8. Design a civil defense plan for a small community.

9. Make sure you know the meanings of warning systems used in your community.

BIBLIOGRAPHY

DEPARTMENT OF DEFENSE, OFFICE OF CIVIL DEFENSE. *In Time of Emergency.* Washington, D. C., 1968.

NATIONAL EDUCATION ASSOCIATION. *Schools and Civil Defense.* Washington, D. C., 1964.

NATIONAL SAFETY COUNCIL. *Accident Facts 1973 Edition.* Chicago, 1973.

———. *Safety in Bad Weather Conditions.* Safety Education Data Sheet No. 76. Chicago, n.d.

NATIONAL SCHOOL BOARDS ASSOCIATION. *School Boards Plan for Civil Defense.* Evanston, Ill., 1965.

OFFICE OF EMERGENCY PREPAREDNESS. *Disaster Preparedness: Report to Congress.* Vols. 1, 2, 3. Washington, D. C., 1972.

13

fire safety

Fire is one of mankind's greatest discoveries. Early man used fire primarily for heating and cooking, and centuries later those are still two of its most important functions. Even today many gourmet cooks claim that using an open flame for broiling meats is a method of cooking that has never been improved upon. The versatility of fire has made man's life more comfortable and convenient. Our daily lives revolve around fire in some form—for cooking, heating, producing electricity, powering automobiles and airplanes, and in the manufacture of innumerable products.

For all its many advantages, however, fire is capable of producing disaster in a matter of seconds. Once out of control, it can ravage a series of buildings, a whole community, a forest, or other valuable property. Conservative estimates place the economic cost of fires in the billions of dollars annually in this country alone. They are also responsible for several thousand deaths each year. In 1972, for example, 6,800 people in the United States died in fires or from burns associated with fires. Of these, 5,700 died in home fires.[1] Figure 13-1 illustrates the ravages of a fire.

Fire has been the cause of many major disasters throughout the United States and the world. On October 9, 1871, a fire almost destroyed the entire city of Chicago and killed nearly 300 people. On that same day,

[1] National Safety Council, *Accident Facts 1973 Edition* (Chicago, 1973), pp. 6, 80.

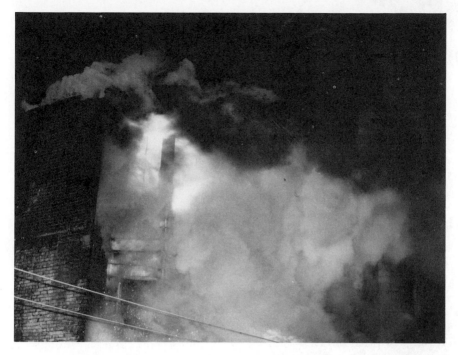

Figure 13-1. A fire in progress. Photo courtesy of Chicago Fire Academy.

a little-publicized fire in Peshtigo, Wisconsin, and the surrounding area killed 1,152 people.[2]

Year in and year out fires continue to take their toll. Ironically a high percentage of these losses could be prevented by using fire prevention principles and common sense rules. Fire is widely recognized as a serious danger, especially when out of control; yet in a highly organized and sophisticated society it is still treated with misapplication and carelessness, as if it were completely harmless.

We understand fire to a great degree. We have the technological knowledge and capability to prevent and retard fires, but we have not been successful in educating people concerning proper use and control. All of us must work to prevent the needless loss of life and destruction from fire.

CAUSES OF FIRES

Non-controlled fires are usually caused by carelessness or failure to apply proper safety precautions. Their cost each year in the number of lives lost

[2] National Safety Council, *Accident Facts 1973*, p. 21.

and the amount of property damage is astronomical. And for the most part, they could be prevented.

electrical fires

An estimated 160,000 electrical fires occur in the United States each year, costing over $270,000,000. Defective wiring, equipment, motors, and power consuming appliances are a major cause. Millions of older homes in America have defective wiring. Most modern homes are equipped with circuit breakers, but many still have fuse boxes. These boxes are often the source of fires when people place coins behind blown fuses or replace the fuses with those of higher amperage than is recommended. A blown fuse indicates a short or an overloaded circuit. When this occurs, the cause should be found. Only appliances and wiring with Underwriters Laboratory approval should be used, and only qualified electricians should make any and all installations.

suspicious, incendiary fires

People with severe personality problems—pyromaniacs, those with revenge or profit motives—purposely start fires. There is no accurate way, however, to determine the actual number of fires occurring from such suspicious causes. Insurance companies are constantly on the lookout for these occurrences. This type of fire is extremely dangerous because it may have a good start before discovery. Estimates put these fires at a cost of over $230,000,000 a year.

heating and cooking equipment

Probably the most dangerous places in the home from the standpoint of fire are the furnace and kitchen areas. Millions of homes also use gas appliances in the form of water heaters, space and central heaters, ranges, grills, and others. When properly used, gas is a valuable service.[3] A misused appliance of any type is unsafe, but gas hazards are unique because of the danger of explosion, as well as asphyxiation, resulting from incomplete combustion. Defective flues or furnaces are a major source of fires. They should be checked annually by qualified people. Heating and cooking equipment is responsible for an estimated 155,000 fires, costing over $170,000,000 each year.

[3] National Safety Council, *Utility Gas in the Home*, Safety Education Data Sheet No. 20 (Chicago, n.d.).

open flames and sparks

Burning rubbish, leaves, boxes, or other items in open areas results in many serious fires—at a cost of over $100,000,000 each year. Adequate fire control equipment with proper precautions should be used when burning leaves or grass. Rubbish should be burned in incinerators constructed for that purpose. Sparks from welding or other equipment are a source of many such fires, as are friction, thawing pipes, and sparks from the embers of other fires.

smoking and matches

Smoking and matches are a major source of fires. Based on 1970 figures of cigarette consumption, if only one out of every three million cigarettes smoked in this country started a fire, there would be a total of 200,000 fires a year from cigarettes alone.[4] Lighted cigarettes generally continue to burn after being carelessly discarded. All cigarettes should be completely extinguished before throwing away. Materials most susceptible to ignition by cigarettes include leaves, paper, and fibers such as cotton. Mattresses and overstuffed furniture are easily ignited—a good reason why absolutely no one should smoke in bed. Many outdoor things such as leaves and rubbish are easily combustible from cigarettes.[5] The improper use of ashtrays and ashtrays of improper construction are also serious fire threats.

wearing apparel

The National Safety Council estimates that 1,500 deaths from clothing fires, as well as 100,000 non-fatal clothing fires, occur annually.[6] Such fires often result in injury to large areas of the body. The burning qualities of different man-made fibers vary considerably. In 1954 Congress passed the Flammable Fabrics Act to protect the public from dangerously flammable wearing apparel hazards. The act was later amended with wider controls. In the event of a clothing fire, do not run, since running fans the flame and accelerates burning. Furthermore, remaining in an upright position allows the flame and smoke to rise upward to the face

---

[4] National Safety Council, *Cigarette Fire Hazards,* Safety Education Data Sheet No. 86 (Chicago, n.d.).

[5] National Safety Council, *Cigarette Fire Hazards.*

[6] National Safety Council, *Flammability of Wearing Apparel,* Safety Education Data Sheet No. 90 (Chicago, n.d.).

and into the lungs. Instead, drop into a horizontal position wherever you are. Remove clothing if possible. If indoors roll a rug or any heavy fabric over yourself. If outdoors roll on the ground. Use anything that can smother or extinguish the flames.[7]

spontaneous ignition

Certain materials such as oily rags or green hay are capable of generating sufficient heat to cause combustion. Oily rags should be disposed of or stored in airtight cans. Farmers should be careful about storing green hay. All newly stored hay should be checked frequently for "hot spots."

Table 13-1 shows the estimated losses in building fires in 1971, categorized both by cause of fire and by occupancy of building.

CHEMISTRY OF COMBUSTION

The National Fire Protection Association defines combustion as:

A chemical process that involves oxygen sufficient to produce light or heat.[8]

Three elements are necessary for combustion to occur: fuel, heat, and oxygen. These elements are what is known as the "fire triangle." When present in the right proportions, they activate the chemical process necessary for a fire. (See Figure 13-2.)

Combustion occurs when fuel molecules and oxygen molecules break down to form intermediate active species, which are called radicals. The radicals react to each other, causing combustion.[9] (See Figure 13-3.)

CLASSES OF FIRES

Fires are classified according to the type of fuel energizing the fire. Knowledge of the classes of fires is important since the type of fuel involved will determine the method of extinguishing the fire. Each class of fire requires a specialized action.

[7] National Safety Council, *Flammability of Wearing Apparel.*
[8] National Fire Protection Association, *Life Safety Code,* NFPA Standard No. 101 (Boston, 1973), p. 7.
[9] Robert F. Wickham, "Clean Agent," *Fire Extinguishing, Environmental and Safety Management Magazine,* October 1970, p. 44.

Table 13-1. Estimated losses in building fires*, 1971.

Cause or Occupancy	No. of Fires	Loss
Totals by Cause..	**996,600**	**$2,266,000,000**
Electrical..	160,900	271,269,000
Wiring and general equipment............................	*98,800*	*188,984,000*
Motors, power-consuming appliances..................	*62,100*	*82,285,000*
Incendiary, suspicious...	72,100	232,947,000
Heating and cooking equipment............................	157,700	172,895,000
Equipment, defective or misused.........................	*87,800*	*111,487,000*
Combustibles near heaters, stoves......................	*39,500*	*41,241,000*
Chimneys, flues defective or overheated.............	*22,400*	*15,862,000*
Hot ashes, coals..	*8,000*	*4,305,000*
Open flames and sparks.......................................	74,100	100,156,000
Welding and cutting torches...............................	*9,700*	*31,497,000*
Sparks from machinery, friction..........................	*16,200*	*19,034,000*
Thawing pipes..	*5,700*	*11,783,000*
Sparks and embers from fires.............................	*5,500*	*5,665,000*
Miscellaneous open flames and sparks...............	*37,000*	*32,177,000*
Smoking and matches..	118,400	98,344,000
Children and matches..	70,400	72,285,000
Flammable liquid fires (not reported elsewhere)......	64,900	53,931,000
Exposure...	23,200	42,148,000
Lightning...	22,200	40,335,000
Spontaneous ignition..	15,700	25,606,000
Rubbish, ignition source unknown.........................	34,400	21,754,000
Gas fires and explosions (not reported elsewhere)...	8,200	21,074,000
Explosions, miscellaneous and unclassified...........	4,400	5,212,000
Miscellaneous known causes...............................	3,800	105,142,000
Unknown or unidentified......................................	166,200	1,002,902,000
Totals by Occupancy.......................................	**996,600**	**$2,266,000,000**
Residential..	699,000	874,100,000
Dwellings, one- and two-family...........................	*536,000*	*608,600,000*
Apartments..	*103,000*	*151,400,000*
Trailers, mobile homes......................................	*25,000*	*36,500,000*
Hotels...	*10,800*	*23,000,000*
Other (motels, rooming houses, summer cottages, etc.)..........	*24,200*	*54,600,000*
Industrial..	41,300	390,000,000
Drugs, chemicals, paints, petroleum...................	*3,100*	*73,700,000*
Metal, metal products.......................................	*3,500*	*45,100,000*
Food products..	*3,700*	*40,200,000*
Mining, mineral products...................................	*1,500*	*39,700,000*
Wood, wood products..	*2,700*	*38,600,000*
Other industrial...	*26,800*	*153,400,000*
Storage...	81,400	358,700,000
Barns and other farm structures.........................	*36,200*	*116,500,000*
Grain elevators..	*3,100*	*49,800,000*
Garages, residential parking..............................	*28,000*	*31,000,000*
Lumber, building material..................................	*1,500*	*21,300,000*
Other storage..	*12,600*	*140,100,000*
Mercantile and office..	71,000	332,200,000
Stores...	*22,100*	*122,600,000*
Motor vehicle sales, repairs and service stations...	*14,400*	*42,600,000*
Offices and banks..	*13,500*	*41,200,000*
Other mercantile..	*21,000*	*125,800,000*
Public assembly and educational..........................	52,200	225,900,000
Schools and colleges.......................................	*20,500*	*87,000,000*
Restaurants, taverns..	*18,200*	*50,900,000*
Theatres, auditoriums, recreation and exhibition halls, etc.....	*4,100*	*27,300,000*
Churches...	*3,400*	*23,300,000*
Other public..	*6,000*	*37,400,000*
Institutional (hospitals, homes for the aged, etc.)...	18,200	22,400,000
Miscellaneous...	33,800	62,200,000

Source: Estimates of National Fire Protection Association.

*Additional nonbuilding fires include: 200 aerospace and aircraft fires with $192,000,000 loss, 111,500 forest fires with $119,000,000 loss, 501,600 motor-vehicle fires with $112,660,000 loss and 42,000 miscellaneous fires with $53,600,000 loss. Totals for building and nonbuilding fires were 1,651,900 fires with $2,743,260,000 loss.

Reproduced from Accident Facts 1973 Edition, *p. 22, courtesy of the National Safety Council.*

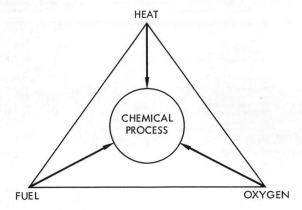

Figure 13-2. The fire triangle.

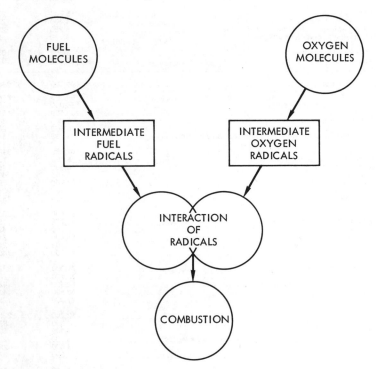

Figure 13-3. The chemistry of combustion.

class A fires

These are fires resulting from the combustion of carbonaceous materials, such as wood and textiles. They are probably the most common type of fire, and the type found in many home fires.

class B fires

These fires result from materials that become gaseous when heated, such as oil, grease and paints.

class C fires

Live electrical equipment is the cause of Class C fires.

class D fires

This specialized classification includes fires from combustible metals, such as magnesium, titanium, zirconium sodium or potassium.

It should be noted that the same fire may involve more than one class as soon as the fire spreads to other materials. Also, once electricity is disconnected, a Class C fire becomes another class of fire.

PRINCIPLES OF EXTINGUISHING FIRES

Based on the principle of the fire triangle, there have long been three ways to extinguish fires: (1) cooling the fuel below its kindling point; (2) excluding the oxygen supply; and (3) separating the fuel from the oxygen. These methods led to the development of different types of extinguishers for different types of fires.

In more recent years new substances, or chemical agents, called halons have been introduced. It is thought that halons interrupt the breakdown in the fuel and oxygen molecules into radicals, which are capable of interacting to cause combustion.[10] This process, however, is not yet fully understood.

Halons belong to the chemical family known as halogens, which are useful as fire extinguishing agents. The halons are identified by number, such as 1211, 1202, 1301, or 2402. The first digit shows the number of carbon atoms present. The second digit signifies the fluorine atoms; the third, chlorine atoms; and the fourth, bromine atoms. Sometimes a fifth digit is used to refer to iodine atoms if present. Of the four potentially useful halons, two are in actual use in the United States—Halon 1301 (the most widely used) and Halon 1211.[11]

[10] Wickham, "Clean Agent," p. 44.

[11] National Safety Council, "Halons (an Evaluation)," *National Safety News*, July 1973, p. 69.

Halon 1301 is an odorless, colorless, electrically non-conductive gas that is effective for all classes of fires. It is a vaporizing agent that leaves no residue, nor does it attack or react with normal materials of construction. Halon 1301 is particularly useful against fires involving delicate electrical, mechanical, or electronic equipment, and high value storage areas such as safes. It has exceptionally low toxicity, and is much safer than any of the vaporizing liquid fire extinguishing agents. Underwriters Laboratories classify Halon 1301 in Group 6 (least toxic).[12] The chief advantages of this agent are personnel safety, versatility against different classes of fires, and cleanliness. Figure 13-4 shows a diagram of a typical Halon 1301 fire-suppression system.

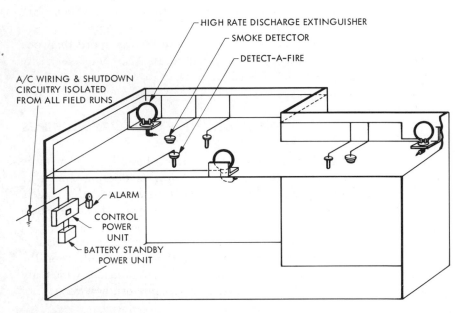

Figure 13-4. A typical Halon 1301 fire suppression system. Courtesy of Fenwal, Inc., Protection Systems Division, Ashland, Mass.

USE OF FIRE EXTINGUISHERS

The type of fire extinguisher used on a specific fire will depend upon the agent that is burning. For example, do not use a fire extinguisher containing water on a grease fire; it will spread the fire and not retard the

[12] Fenwal, Inc., Protection Systems Division, *Halon 1301 Fire Suppression System: Installation, Operation and Maintenance Manual* (Ashland, Mass., 1973), p. 3.

flame. The water extinguisher would also not be useful in an electrical fire; water conducts electricity, thus becoming hazardous for the operator.

For Class A fires (wood and papers), extinguishers containing water, which will cool and quench the burning material, are suitable. Dry chemical extinguishers may also be used since they provide a fire retardant blanket to prevent reflash.

For Class B fires (oils, greases, paints), carbon dioxide extinguishers are excellent. Carbon dioxide leaves no residue and will not affect equipment or foodstuffs. Dry chemical extinguishers are also useful in these fires.

For Class C fires (electrical equipment), use either a carbon dioxide extinguisher (carbon dioxide is non-conductive) or a dry chemical extinguisher. Dry chemical extinguishers are called tri-class extinguishers since they can be used on Class A, B, and C fires.

For Class D fires (combustible metals), special extinguishing powders may be applied by a scoop or shovel.

Figure 13-5 shows a demonstration of the proper technique in using a fire extinguisher.

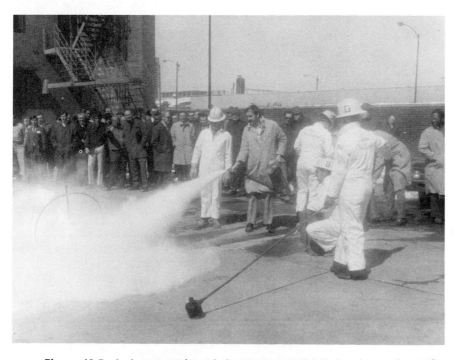

Figure 13-5. A demonstration of the correct method of using a fire extinguisher. Photo courtesy of Chicago Fire Academy.

identification of fire extinguishers

Since an incorrect material on a specific fire can do more harm than good, and may actually be dangerous, it is important that fire extinguishers be well marked for quick identification under emergency conditions. In the excitement of a fire it is very easy to grab the wrong type of extinguisher. Before using any extinguisher, a person should read the labels. Usually fire extinguishers are marked with decals, paintings, or similar methods. Sometimes wall panel markings are used near the extinguisher for identification purposes. Markings on extinguishers should be durable, with easy legibility at a distance of 3 feet. Wall markings should be legible from a distance of 25 feet.[13]

The National Fire Protection Association recommends the following markings for various extinguishers:

1. Extinguishers suitable for use on Class A fires should be identified by a triangle containing the letter "A." If the triangle is colored, it should be colored green.
2. Extinguishers suitable for use on Class B fires should be identified by a square containing the letter "B." If the square is colored, it should be colored red.
3. Class C fire extinguishers should be identified by a circle containing the letter "C." If colored, the circle should be colored blue.
4. Extinguishers suitable for fires involving metals should be identified by a five-pointed star that contains the letter "D." If the star is colored, it should be yellow.

Extinguishers suitable for more than one class of fire may be identified by multiple symbols.[14] Figure 13-6 shows typical fire extinguisher markings in use today.

All fire extinguishers, whether in homes, industry, or elsewhere, should be checked frequently to be sure they are in working order. One should determine if the extinguishers are full and whether they have been tampered with. Proper maintenance, including checking for needed repairs, recharging or replacement, should be carried out annually. Maintenance is more than a quick check.

Factories, offices, shops, schools, churches, and homes should be

[13] National Fire Protection Association, *Installation of Portable Fire Extinguishers 1973*, NFPA Standard No. 10 (Boston, 1973), p. 33.
[14] National Fire Protection Association, *Installation of Fire Extinguishers*, p. 33.

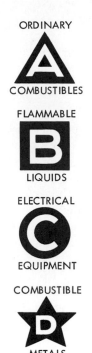

ORDINARY

A

COMBUSTIBLES

FLAMMABLE

B

LIQUIDS

ELECTRICAL

C

EQUIPMENT

COMBUSTIBLE

D

METALS

Figure 13-6. Fire extinguisher markings. Courtesy of National Fire Protection Association.

surveyed by experts to determine the type of fire protection equipment needed, including the placement of extinguishers. Several factors will determine selection and placement, but generally they should be placed in accordance with the type and size of fire that can be anticipated in a given area.

The National Fire Protection Association classifies rooms in a general manner according to the type and amount of hazard present:

1. Light Hazards. Where the amount of combustibles or flammable liquids present is such that fires of small size may be expected. These may include offices, schoolrooms, churches, assembly halls, telephone exchanges, etc.
2. Ordinary Hazards. Where the amount of combustibles or flammable liquids present is such that fires of moderate size may be expected. These may include mercantile storage and display, auto showrooms, parking garages, light manufacturing, warehouses not classified as extra hazards, school shop areas, etc.
3. Extra Hazards. Where the amount of combustibles or flammable liquids present is such that fires of severe magnitude may be expected. These may include woodworking, auto repair, aircraft servicing, ware-

houses with high-piled (over 15 feet in solid piles, over 12 feet in piles that contain no horizontal channels) combustibles, and processes such as flammable liquid handling, painting, dipping, etc.[15]

SUMMARY

Fire is one of man's greatest servants and one of his greatest threats. A huge percentage of fire deaths and property losses could be prevented if people would take proper precautions and use our present technological knowledge against fire.

The high number of fires, the excessive losses in lives and property epitomize our lack of education in fire prevention. Somewhere we are failing badly in an area where we have the ability and knowledge for almost complete protection. Schools and other agencies must do more in fire protection education.

Fire prevention and fire fighting are sciences based on our knowledge of fire chemistry. All industries, businesses, public places, and homes should make surveys to determine the existing hazards and methods for compensating for them. Fire departments will cooperate.

SUGGESTED STUDENT ACTIVITIES

1. Check the fire extinguishers in your school and community to determine when they were serviced last or if they have been tampered with.
2. Visit your fire department and ascertain the number and if possible the estimated costs of fires in your local community during the past five years. Prepare graphs of these statistics to indicate trends.
3. Write a paper on arson and pyromania. Illustrate how fire investigators determine if arson occurred.
4. Visit an insurance office. Determine their criteria for insuring a school or factory against fire losses.
5. Survey your school building for fire hazards.
6. Survey your home and plan a method of escape that can be executed by your family in the event of fire.

BIBLIOGRAPHY

FENWAL, INC., PROTECTION SYSTEMS DIVISION. *Halon 1301 Fire Suppression System: Installation, Operation and Maintenance Manual.* Ashland, Mass., 1973.

[15] National Fire Protection Association, *Installation of Fire Extinguishers*, p. 15.

NATIONAL FIRE PROTECTION ASSOCIATION. *Installation of Portable Fire Extinguishers 1973.* NFPA Standard No. 10. Boston, 1973.

————. *Life Safety Code.* NFPA Standard No. 101. Boston, 1973.

NATIONAL SAFETY COUNCIL. *Accident Facts 1973 Edition.* Chicago, 1973.

————. *Cigarette Fire Hazards.* Safety Education Data Sheet No. 86. Chicago, n.d.

————. *Flammability of Wearing Apparel.* Safety Education Data Sheet No. 90. Chicago, n.d.

————. "Halons (an Evaluation)." *National Safety News,* July 1973, p. 69.

————. *Utility Gas in the Home.* Safety Education Data Sheet No. 20. Chicago, n.d.

WICKHAM, ROBERT F. "Clean Agent." *Fire Extinguishing, Environmental and Safety Management Magazine,* October 1970, p. 44.

14

safety as a
professional career

Safety is a multi-discipline profession, drawing its workers from many different areas—education, engineering, psychology, medicine, biophysics, and so forth. Many of these people have already made valuable contributions in the field of accident prevention. Interestingly, many workers in the field did not actually choose safety as a profession, but instead became interested in accident prevention while working in their own areas. The fact that a profession could develop in this manner is evidence of the universal interest in safety by all people. Figure 14-1 illustrates some of the specialties involved in safety work.

Compared to law, engineering, medicine, dentistry, or education, the safety profession is very young. It has been recognized as a true profession only in recent years. Almost anyone could be put in charge of safety programs years ago, but today the true safety professional is emerging, with strict standards for certification, and programs are being developed to meet the needs of various types of safety personnel.

Today the need for safety professionals is evidenced by the growth in the number of people engaged full time in some phase of safety, whether in education, industry, traffic, or elsewhere. Recent federal legislation has placed much emphasis on the safety movement, and safety as a profession should make great strides in accident prevention and in the upgrading of the profession itself.

Millions of people also work part time in some phase of safety. The policeman directing traffic, the elementary teacher or the driver education

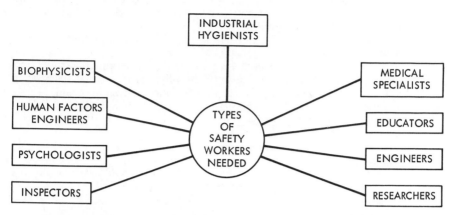

Figure 14-1. *A partial listing of some of the specialists needed for safety work.*

teacher presenting a lesson, the industrial engineer or the industrial hygienist eliminating a hazard in industry, and the psychologist studying human behavior are all performing safety functions.

Many organizations, such as the National Safety Council, the American Society of Safety Engineers, the American Automobile Association, the American Driver Education and Traffic Education Association, and many others, have helped to promulgate standards for the certification of safety workers. Safety has arrived as a true profession.

THE SCOPE AND FUNCTION OF THE PROFESSIONAL SAFETY POSITION

Note: This section is a reprint of a brochure prepared by the American Society of Safety Engineers, and is reprinted courtesy of the Society.[1]

The Scope of the Professional Safety Position

The safety professional brings together those elements of the various disciplines necessary to identify and evaluate the magnitude of the safety problem. He collects and analyzes the information essential to the solution of the problem. He is concerned with all facets of the problem, personal and environmental, transient and permanent, to determine the causes of accidents or the existence of loss producing conditions, practices or materials.

[1] American Society of Safety Engineers, *Scope and Function of the Professional Safety Position*, special publication (Park Ridge, Ill., n.d.).

Based upon the information he has collected and analyzed, he proposes alternate solutions, together with recommendations based upon his specialized knowledge and experience, to those who have ultimate decision-making responsibilities.

The functions of the position are described as they may be applied in principle to the safety professional in any activity.

The safety professional in performing these functions will draw upon specialized knowledge in both the physical and social sciences. He will apply the principles of measurement and analysis to evaluate safety performance. He will be required to have fundamental knowledge of statistics, mathematics, physics, chemistry, as well as the fundamentals of the engineering disciplines.

He will utilize knowledge in the fields of behavior, motivation, and communications. Knowledge of management principles as well as the theory of business and government organization will also be required. His specialized knowledge must include a thorough understanding of the causative factors contributing to accident occurrence as well as methods and procedures designed to control such events.

The safety professional of the future will need a unique and diversified type of education and training if he is to meet the challenges of the future. The population explosion, the problems of urban areas, future transportation systems, as well as the increasing complexities of man's every day life will create many problems and extend the safety professional's creativity to its maximum if he is to successfully provide the knowledge and leadership to conserve life, health and property.

Functions of the Professional Safety Position

The major functions of the safety professional are contained within four basic areas. However, application of all or some of the functions listed below will depend upon the nature and scope of the existing accident problems, and the type of activity with which he is concerned.

The major areas are:

A. Identification and appraisal of accident and loss producing conditions and practices and evaluation of the severity of the accident problem.
B. Development of accident prevention and loss control methods, procedures, and programs.
C. Communication of accident and loss control information to those directly involved.
D. Measurement and evaluation of the effectiveness of the accident and loss control system and the modifications needed to achieve optimum results.

A. Identification and Appraisal of Accident and Loss Producing Conditions and Practices and Evaluation of the Severity of the Accident Problem

These functions involve:

1. The development of methods of identifying hazards and evaluating the loss producing potential of a given system, operation or process by:
   a. Advanced detailed studies of hazards of planned and proposed facilities, operations and products.
   b. Hazard analysis of existing facilities, operations and products.
2. The preparation and interpretation of analyses of the total economic loss resulting from the accident and losses under consideration.

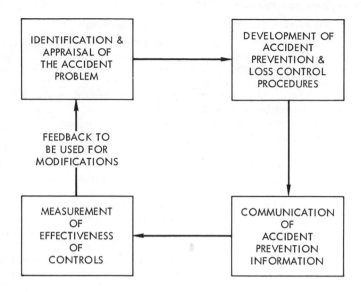

3. The review of the entire system in detail to define likely modes of failure, including human error and their effects on the safety of the system.
   a. The identification of errors involving incomplete decision making, faulty judgment, administrative miscalculation and poor practices.
   b. The designation of potential weaknesses found in existing policies, directives, objectives, or practices.
4. The review of reports of injuries, property damage, occupational diseases or public liability accidents and the compilation, analysis and interpretation of relevant causative factor information.
   a. The establishment of a classification system that will make it possible to identify significant causative factors and determine trends.
   b. The establishment of a system to insure the completeness and validity of the reported information.
   c. The conduct of thorough investigation of those accidents where specialized knowledge and skill are required.
5. The provision of advice and counsel concerning compliance with applicable laws, codes, regulations and standards.
6. The conduct of research studies of technical safety problems.
7. The determination of the need of surveys and appraisals by related specialists such as medical, health physicists, industrial hygienists, fire protection engineers and psychologists to identify conditions affecting the health and safety of individuals.
8. The systematic study of the various elements of the environment to assure that tasks and exposures of the individual are within his psychological and physiological limitations and capacities.

B. Development of Accident Prevention and Loss Control Methods, Procedures and Programs

In carrying out this function, the safety professional:

1. Uses his specialized knowledge of accident causation and control to prescribe an integrated accident and loss control system designed to:
    a. Eliminate causative factors associated with the accident problem, preferably before an accident occurs.
    b. Where it is not possible to eliminate the hazard, devise mechanisms to reduce the degree of hazard.
    c. Reduce the severity of the results of an accident by prescribing specialized equipment designed to reduce the severity of an injury should an accident occur.
2. Establishes methods to demonstrate the relationship of safety performance to the primary function of the entire operation or any of its components.
3. Develops policies, codes, safety standards and procedures that become part of the operational policies of the organization.
4. Incorporates essential safety and health requirements in all purchasing and contracting specifications.
5. As a professional safety consultant for personnel engaged in planning, design, development, installation of various parts of the system, advises and consults on the necessary modification to insure consideration of all potential hazards.
6. Coordinates the results of job analysis to assist in proper selection and placement of personnel, whose capabilities and/or limitations are suited to the operation involved.
7. Consults concerning product safety, including the intended and potential uses of the product as well as its material and construction, through the establishment of general requirements for the application of safety principles throughout planning, design, development, fabrication and test of various products, to achieve maximum product safety.
8. Systematically reviews technological developments and equipment to keep up to date on the devices and techniques designed to eliminate or minimize hazards, and determine whether these developments and techniques have any applications to the activities with which he is concerned.

C. Communication of Accident and Loss Control Information to those Directly Involved

In carrying out this function the safety professional:

1. Compiles, analyzes and interprets accident statistical data and prepares reports designed to communicate this information to those personnel concerned.
2. Communicates recommended controls, procedures, or programs, designed to eliminate or minimize hazard potential, to the appropriate person or persons.
3. Through appropriate communication media, persuades those who have ultimate decision making responsibilities to adopt and utilize those controls which the preponderance of evidence indicates are best suited to achieve the desired results.

4. Directs or assists in the development of specialized education and training materials and in the conduct of specialized training programs for those who have operational responsibility.
5. Provides advice and counsel on the type and channels of communications to insure the timely and efficient transmission of useable accident prevention information to those concerned.

D. Measurement and Evaluation of the Effectiveness of the Accident and Loss Control System and the Needed Modifications to Achieve Optimum Results

1. Establishes measurement techniques such as cost statistics, work sampling or other appropriate means, for obtaining periodic and systematic evaluation of the effectiveness of the control system.
2. Develops methods that will evaluate the costs of the control system in terms of the effectiveness of each part of the system and its contribution to accident and loss reduction.
3. Provides feed back information concerning the effectiveness of the control measures to those with ultimate responsibility, with the recommended adjustments or changes as indicated by the analyses.

JOB OPPORTUNITIES IN THE SAFETY PROFESSION

The three major employers of safety personnel are the government (all levels), private industry, and insurance companies.[2] Private consulting firms specializing in safety functions, such as loss control or traffic safety engineering, also employ safety professionals. In addition, many professional and private organizations, such as associations, safety councils, and unions, are a source of job opportunities. There are thousands of driver education teachers in the nation's public and private schools, and thousands more employed in commercial driving schools. Figures 14-2 and 14-3 show a partial listing of private and governmental organizations that employ safety personnel.

There is presently a shortage of well-trained workers in practically all phases of safety. We can expect this trend to continue with the extension of legislation in occupational safety, product safety, and environmental health. Growth in the trade and service industries and the expanding safety needs of educational institutions, construction, transportation, insurance and governmental groups should further accentuate the demand for safety workers.[3]

A recent estimate places the shortage in occupational safety and health manpower at 5,000 to 10,000 safety professionals, 10,000 industrial

[2] William J. Killen, "Safety Career Opportunities," *Environmental Control and Safety Management,* August 1071, p. 12.
[3] American Society of Safety Engineers, *Demand for Safety Personnel,* special bulletin (Park Ridge, Ill., 1973), p. 1.

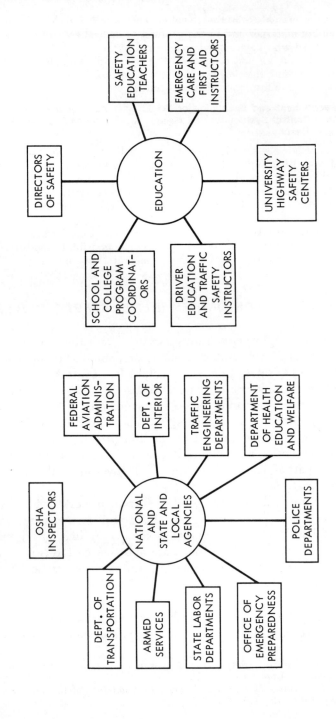

Figure 14-2. *Governmental and educational employment opportunities in safety. Note: the charts do not include all government agencies which employ safety personnel.*

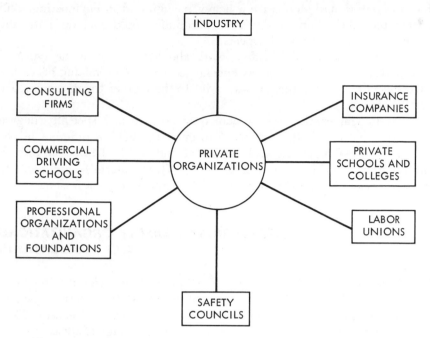

Figure 14-3. Private sources of employment opportunities in safety.

hygienists, 3,000 occupational health physicians, 10,000 occupational health nurses, and 8,000 occupational health scientists.[4]

All of this points to a bright future for those who are willing to acquire the necessary education and experience. Corporate safety directors and many others with lesser responsibilities enjoy excellent salaries. In fact the pay scale for most safety workers is excellent.

Obviously, there is a need in safety work for people with varying degrees of education and experience. The range of opportunities extends from what could be considered para-professional to the highly trained and skilled individual at the corporate management level, and includes safety educators and government safety inspectors and researchers.

The type of training needed will, of course, depend on the individual job requirements, which presents some difficulties for those preparing to enter the health and safety occupations. Some authorities view the health and safety specialist as a behaviorist and would therefore direct his or her training toward the behavioral sciences, such as psychology. Others see the specialist as a technician able to handle the technical problems of

---

[4] Edgar F. Seagle, "Opportunities for Safety Education," *National Safety News,* January 1972, p. 58.

hazard control, and emphasize a heavy background in engineering. Still others feel the safety worker's background should include both the engineering and behavioral aspects.[5]

Anyone interested in safety work should investigate the types of jobs performed by various safety specialists before determining his or her own specialty. This in turn should indicate the type of training necessary for the chosen area.

Many universities offer a choice of courses and specialty degree programs that enable the individual to enter the field at different levels. The professional organizations listed at the end of this chapter can furnish information concerning university and college offerings pertinent to various specialties and levels of entry into the safety profession.

PROFESSIONAL SAFETY ORGANIZATIONS AND PUBLICATIONS

The formation of professional organizations and agencies is direct evidence that a discipline is acquiring professional status. These organizations are formed for the purpose of promoting professional causes. They provide excellent vehicles for research, for the exchange of ideas, and for the upgrading of standards within the profession. One of the earliest and most influential in the field of safety is the American Society of Safety Engineers, founded in 1911 as the United Association of Casualty Inspectors and forerunner of the National Safety Council. The ASSE now has approximately 12,000 members employed in all areas of the economy. Its objective is:

> To promote the advancement of the profession and contribute to the well-being and professional development of its members.[6]

Several other organizations are vitally interested in safety. They include the Institute of Traffic Engineers, in the area of traffic engineering and traffic safety, and the National Board of Fire Underwriters, which is interested in fire safety.

Professional organizations publish periodicals, magazines, and other safety materials, providing their membership with up-to-date information

[5] Robert J. Firenze, "A Bachelor's Degree in Industrial Safety," *National Safety News*, June 1972, p. 53.
[6] American Society of Safety Engineers, *Position Statement: Qualifications of Occupational Safety and Health Personnel in Governmental Programs*, special publication (Park Ridge, Ill., 1973).

on what is happening within the profession. Many of the organizations supply information on job opportunities in the field.

The National Safety Council reports over 40 safety centers in the United States that are located in universities or colleges. These centers have varied educational programs in such fields as education, traffic, general safety, and in some cases police training. Their overall purpose is to solve safety problems by coordinating multi-disciplinary efforts in education and training, public service, and research.[7]

Following is a partial listing of the major organizations promoting safety in the United States. Also included is a list of publications sponsored by some of the organizations. These lists are by no means comprehensive, so not all of the excellent organizations or publications are listed.

professional organizations

American Association for Health,
Physical Education, and Recreation
1201 16th Street, N.W.
Washington, D. C. 20036

American Automobile
Association
8111 Gatehouse Road
Falls Church, Va. 22042

American Medical Association
535 North Dearborn
Chicago, Ill. 60610

American Society of Safety
Engineers
850 Busse Highway
Park Ridge, Ill. 60068

Institute of Traffic Engineers
1815 North Ft. Myers Drive
Suite 905
Arlington, Va. 22209

American Association of
Motor Vehicle Administrators
1828 L. Street, N.W.
Suite 500
Washington, D. C. 20036

American Driver and Traffic
Education Association
1201 16th Street, N.W.
Washington, D. C. 20036

American School Health
Association
Kent, Ohio 44240

Eno Foundation for
Transportation
Westport, Conn. 06880

Insurance Institute for
Highway Safety
Watergate 600
Washington, D. C. 20037

[7] National Safety Council, *College and University Highway Traffic and Safety Centers,* special publication, College and University Safety Center Division (Chicago, n.d.).

National Education Association
1201 16th Street, N.W.
Washington, D. C. 20036

National Highway Traffic
Safety Administration
U.S. Department of
Transportation
Washington, D. C. 20590

Occupational Safety and
Health Administration
U.S. Department of Labor
1726 M. Street, N.W.
Washington, D. C. 20210

Safe Winter Driving League
625 North Michigan Avenue
Chicago, Ill. 60611

National Fire Protection
Association
470 Atlantic Avenue
Boston, Mass. 02210

National Safety Council
425 North Michigan Avenue
Chicago, Ill. 60611

Public Safety Institute
The Pennsylvania State
University
University City, Pa. 16801

Underwriters Laboratories, Inc.
207 West Ohio Street
Chicago, Ill. 60611

safety periodicals

PUBLISHING ORGANIZATION	TITLE	SEQUENCE
Aetna Life and Casualty 151 Farmington Avenue Hartford, Conn. 06115	*Concepts*	Quarterly
Allstate Insurance Allstate Plaza Northbrook, Ill. 60062	*Analogy*	Quarterly
American Society of Safety Engineers 850 Busse Highway Park Ridge, Ill. 60058	*Journal of American Society of Safety Engineers*	Monthly
Behavioral Publications 2852 Broadway Morningside Heights New York, N. Y. 10025	*Behavioral Research in Highway Safety*	Quarterly
California Driver Education Association 413 Dahlia Corona del Mar, Calif. 92625	*Journal of Traffic Safety Education*	Bi-monthly except summer months

Eno Foundation for Transportation Westport, Conn. 06880	*Traffic Quarterly*	Quarterly
Institute of Traffic Engineers 1815 N. Fort Myers Drive Arlington, Va. 22209	*Traffic Engineering*	Monthly
Metropolitan Life Insurance Co. One Madison Avenue New York, N. Y. 10010	*Statistical Bulletin*	Monthly
National Safety Council 425 North Michigan Avenue Chicago, Ill. 60611	*Family Safety*	Quarterly
	Farm Safety Review	Bi-monthly
	Industrial Supervisor	Monthly
	Journal of Safety Research	Quarterly
	National Safety Congress Transactions	Annually
	National Safety News	Monthly
	Teaching About Safety	Quarterly
	Traffic Safety	Monthly
	Various Departmental Newsletters	
Traffic Institute Northwestern University 1804 Hinman Avenue Evanston, Ill. 60204	*Traffic Digest and Review*	Monthly

SUMMARY

The outlook for job opportunities in the health and safety profession is excellent. An existing shortage of workers in the field will be increased by federal legislation in the area of occupational safety, product safety, and environmental health.

The profession is multi-disciplined, offering opportunities for people from different walks of life. One should closely examine the different job opportunities and plan his or her education to qualify for a job in the field of particular interest.

The profession has arrived as a "profession." We can reasonably expect more sophisticated research and a general upgrading of standards for certification of safety workers. Working in the profession is a very satisfying experience—a safety worker must be one who enjoys helping others. An adage for those preparing for work in the field might be, "The only thing that is more expensive than education is lack of education." Those entering the safety field today have almost unlimited possibilities.

SUGGESTED STUDENT ACTIVITIES

1. Write a paper proposing an educational curriculum for preparing people in a given specialty in the safety field.
2. Examine the curricula of two different colleges offering degree programs in safety. Determine the difference.
3. Invite a safety professional to speak before your class and explain the scope of his duties.
4. Prepare a graph showing the pay levels of various safety jobs.
5. Write a job description and prepare a task analysis for a safety supervisor.

BIBLIOGRAPHY

AMERICAN SOCIETY OF SAFETY ENGINEERS. *The Demand for Safety Personnel.* Special bulletin. Park Ridge, Ill., 1973.

————. *Position Statement: Qualifications of Occupational Safety and Health Personnel in Governmental Programs.* Special publication. Park Ridge, Ill., 1973.

————. *Scope and Function of the Professional Safety Position.* Special publication. Park Ridge, Ill., n.d.

FIRENZE, ROBERT J. "A Bachelor's Degree in Industrial Safety." *National Safety News,* June 1972, p. 53.

KILLEN, WILLIAM J. "Safety Career Opportunities." *Environmental Control and Safety Management,* August 1971, p. 12.

NATIONAL SAFETY COUNCIL. *College and University Highway Traffic and Safety Centers.* Special publication, College and University Safety Center Division. Chicago, n.d.

SEAGLE, EDGAR F. "Opportunities for Safety Education." *National Safety News,* January 1972, p. 58.

15

problems in accident research

Research is a method of inquiry used to find answers to man's problems. In all areas of life there is a positive relationship between man's progress and the success of his research efforts. In recent years our more progressive research programs have produced dramatic advances—polio vaccine, antibiotic drugs, supersonic jets, automated equipment, and men on the moon, to name only a few.

To join in this success, accident research will have to do two things: determine the causes of accidents; and develop effective countermeasures to prevent them.

GENERAL PROBLEMS OF ACCIDENT RESEARCH

Accident research is not unique in the number of its problems nor in the elusiveness of their answers. One major problem that impedes accident research is lack of public support. The public simply does not get overly concerned about accidents. Yet the research programs that attract large sums of money and the best talent must have considerable public support. Society's aims and goals have to be reevaluated.

Most authorities feel that the nature of accidents themselves is largely responsible for public apathy. Except for a dramatic airplane crash or the like, people do not give accidents the same attention as an epidemic or a race to the moon. Instead, they are regarded as isolated events. But isolated or not, accidents accumulate massive totals in deaths, injuries, and property losses. It seems incredible, although true, that people are apathetic to what is the fourth largest killer among all age groups and the leading killer among the 0–38-year-olds.

Another major reason for public apathy is that people tend to see accidents as chance events occurring in random fashion. If they are chance events, then there is really not very much that a person can do about them. If I'm lucky, people reason, an accident won't happen to me. If I'm not, I can't prevent it anyway. And yet investigation has shown that most accidents are *not* chance events; they are caused. And if accidents are caused, then something can indeed be done to stop them. The public must be educated to change the way in which it regards accidents. Only then will people do something about preventing them.

Safety workers have been largely unsuccessful in their efforts to reeducate the public with such slogans as "Safety first" and "The life you save may be your own." However, society does respond to causes. This was proven by the polio foundation, which effectively dramatized a problem far less significant in terms of numbers than accidents. Other research programs have also been successful in arousing public support. People have acknowledged that some problems do warrant the necessary efforts and expenditures. We must reevaluate, redesign, and specifically target our educational programs concerning accidents. If and when society places accidents into proper perspective, it will undoubtedly provide the impetus necessary to improve all efforts in accident prevention, including research.

The characteristics of accidents themselves make the collection and collation of useful accident data extremely difficult. No research program can be generated or sustained without adequate and valid data. Accidents are the terminal event in a sequence of events that produce injury, death, or property damage. This means in many cases that the accidents are not observed. It also means that the investigation must work backward from the terminal event to determine the sequence of events leading up to the accident. Although many of the proximate causes will be obvious, many casual but important factors may be obscure. We must then consider the accident and the system in which it occurred and not just the accident itself.

Our present systems of collecting accident data fail to collect all the information necessary to determine all proximate and casual causes. It therefore becomes difficult, if not impossible, to assign meaningful weights to the variables in individual accidents and even more difficult to apply the variables to groups of accidents.

Industry has had the most success in accident data collection, as reflected in the success of their accident prevention programs. In fact, industry represents the brightest spot in accident prevention. This is especially true of the larger, more progressive, and well-organized industries. Federal legislation (OSHA) should further promote these efforts in industry, especially among the smaller and less well-organized industries. This legislation requires good accident reporting systems and provides standards for accident reporting forms and reporting systems.

The most reliable source of general accident frequency data is the National Safety Council. It collects the data from many sources and disseminates it annually in a publication known as *Accident Facts* which provides a good overview of the entire accident problem. The accidents are classified in several ways, such as type of accident and place of occurrence. Such variables as sex, age, and time of day are included in many of the classifications. This publication highlights the accident problem. It stresses the need for certain priority actions in accident prevention. For example, it points out that auto accidents and home accidents need immediate and special attention, without demeaning the importance of accidents in other areas.

Another stumbling block to accident investigation is the inability of authorities to agree on how to define an accident. Definitions enable us to delimit research and promote general agreement. Edward A. Suchman says that we would be better to list a set of events that characterize accidents than to attempt to define accidents as a single unitary concept.[1] He lists the following major characteristics that might be used in defining an accident:

1. Degree of expectedness—the less the event could have been anticipated, the more likely it is to be labeled an accident.
2. Degree of avoidability—the less the event could have been avoided, the more likely it is to be labeled an accident.
3. Degree of intention—the less the event was the result of deliberate action, the more likely it is to be labeled an accident.[2]

According to Suchman, this approach would define accidents as a class of events involving a low level of expectedness, of avoidability, and of intention. Therefore, in addition to those events that result in bodily injury (such as medical accidents), he would include such unexpected, unavoidable, and unintentional acts as losing things, or forgetting appointments.[3]

---

[1] Edward A. Suchman, "A Conceptual Analysis of the Accident Phenomenon," in *Behavioral Approaches to Accident Research,* Association for the Aid of Crippled Children (New York: Canis and Harris, 1961), p. 00.

[2] Suchman, "The Accident Phenomenon," pp. 30–31.

[3] Suchman, "The Accident Phenomenon," p. 31.

Regardless of what definition is finally chosen, there must be some agreement on what constitutes an accident. Researchers must give more attention to defining all terms more accurately so that others may understand exactly the confines within which they are working.

Other serious problems related to accident research are such things as:

1. Lack of well-trained investigators.
2. Lack of bonafide safety centers with proper equipment and properly trained personnel.
3. Lack of funds resulting from poor public support.
4. Lack of sophistication in the adoption, application, and evaluation of countermeasure programs.

CURRENT STATUS OF ACCIDENT RESEARCH

The low status of accident research is reflected in its problems. How have the symptoms of these problems shown themselves in the current accident research picture? Generally speaking, the results are poorly designed research projects with a wide range of quantitative and qualitative results. Obviously, we would be much better off with more quality and less quantity. From a professional standpoint, much of the research has been low keyed. Dr. Gerald Driessen of the National Safety Council, referring specifically to research in driver education, described the total accident research picture in this way:

> Criticizing the design of experimental studies in the area of driver education is as easy as walking downhill. Things are in terrible shape.[4]

The shortage of trained researchers has contributed heavily to the problem. The result has been the proliferation of research based on insufficient and inaccurate data, poor use of control groups, and lack of consideration of such things as exposure.

Due to weaknesses in methodology and control, much of this research has produced numerous erroneous conclusions. In many cases these wrong conclusions have shifted attention in the wrong direction and created confusion in the entire accident research picture. Such a situation tends to dissipate badly needed funds.

In many areas, however, we have had very good research. For

[4] Gerald Driessen, "The Fallacy of the Untrained Driver," *Traffic Safety Magazine,* March 1969, p. 17.

example, excellent safety devices and hardware are the result of highly sophisticated research conducted by well-trained scientists. For the most part, this research has been carried out in the larger industries, such as automobile and aircraft manufacturing.

The aerospace industry uses systems analysis techniques. These techniques are spreading, and in the future safety professionals will hear much more about systems safety.[5] The systems philosophy recognizes that man is operating in a complex environment containing many machines and other agents. Systems analysis techniques represent the most promising innovation in the safety field in many years.

Some universities, professional organizations, government agencies, and others have sponsored much fine research. In the area of human behavior, for example, a number of useful studies have originated from controlled laboratories.

Excellent research has been carried out on the effects of alcohol on driving. It has given proper consideration to exposure elements and also has carefully delimited its findings. Research in the agricultural industry has also given consideration to exposure. (Ironically, although there is probably much valid research already completed and probably much more underway, the lack of communication among safety professionals tends to keep the results of such studies beyond the reach of the profession in general.)

Even with some bright spots, the picture badly needs improvement. Basically the problem is that we have no organization where research efforts can be centralized. As a result, research is not well classified and delimited. It has unnecessary duplication; it needs better methodology, better control, and better direction. Every effort should be made to reduce the number of accidents and their consequences as fast as possible.

RECOMMENDATIONS FOR FUTURE ACCIDENT RESEARCH

The complex problem of determining the origin of accidents permeates all levels of accident investigation. The scope and diversity of problems in accident research indicate a need for a balanced approach involving many disciplines, such as medicine, psychology, sociology, biophysics, biostatistics, and engineering. William Haddon, Edward Suchman, and David Klein expressed the need for a balanced approach in this way:

[5] J. L. Recht, *Systems Safety Analysis: A Modern Approach to Safety Problems,* special publication (Chicago: National Safety Council, n.d.), p. 1.

Ideally the approach must be intentionally multifactoral and must avoid presuppositions as to the primary causes either of accidents in general or of those in the specific group under study.[6]

We need research into the scope of accident investigation itself.[7] Special attention should be given to methods, balance, and ways of coordinating all accident research. None of the various fields or disciplines is mutually exclusive of each other. The discovery of the polio vaccine is a good example of a balanced research approach. Without question Dr. Jonas Salk is a brilliant researcher. However, part of his success in this historical achievement was due to his willingness and ability to examine the work of others, as well as his own, and to piece a jigsaw puzzle together.

The importance of almost unlimited research promoted by the National Foundation for Infantile Paralysis (now the National Foundation) is due in large part to its outstanding coordination. The same type of orderly, well-organized approach would greatly facilitate accident investigation.

Where does one begin to bring about such a coordinated effort? There are many private, professional, and government organizations interested in accident research. Obviously, one of these groups must exercise the leadership. At present the most logical organization would probably be the National Safety Council or the federal government.

Whichever organization assumes the leadership, it will need the cooperation and assistance of all safety oriented organizations in the country for initial financing and other matters. Its first step should be a careful survey of the nature and scope of past and present research to assess where we are now in terms of completed and needed future research.

The second step would be to decide on a classification system for accident research and a workable arrangement for coordinating future research, based on needs as indicated by research into present programs. Although the eventual shape of such a program cannot be predicted at this time, one possible method of classifying accident research problem areas is shown in the following outline:

ACCIDENT RESEARCH PROBLEM AREAS

I. Accident Causation (and Severity) Research
   A. Investigation and Analysis of Individual Accidents

[6] William Haddon, Jr., Edward A. Suchman, and David Klein, *Accident Research, Methods and Approaches*, Association for the Aid of Crippled Children (New York: Harper & Row, 1964), p. 15.
[7] B. G. King, "Some Comments on Accident Prevention Research," *Traffic Safety Research Review* 7 (June 1963), pp. 19–21.

   B. Investigation of Accidents Classified by Risk Situation
   C. Investigation of Accident-generating Individuals, Situations, or
       Processes

  II. Accident Prevention Research
   A. Countermeasure Development Research
   B. Countermeasure Effectiveness Evaluation
   C. Countermeasure Acceptability Evaluation

 III. Accident-related Behavioral Research
   A. General Behavioral Process
       Examples: Risk Perception
                 Risk Taking
                 Learning
                 Relative Motion Perception
                 Attitude Formation
   B. Specific Behavioral Processes
       Examples: Driving Behavior
                 Drinking Behavior
                 Formation of Attitudes Toward Safety [8]

   After the kind of organizational apparatus is finally determined, a
national research center should be established and organized to meet
the desired objectives. This center should serve as the focal point for
coordination of research carried on in a national network of subcenters
specializing in certain types of research compatible with the overall
accident research program. Figure 15-1 shows how the organization chart
for a network of research centers might appear.
   This would eliminate much duplication of research and reduce the
unnecessary dissipation of needed funds. The goal should be to reduce
all accidents to an irreducible minimum as quickly as possible. A well-
coordinated team effort would certainly achieve this goal much faster
than our present method, in which the left hand does not know what
the right hand is doing. Figure 15-2 shows a model of how a coordinated
research project might work in a given center. A system of this type
would permit the pooling of the best minds in the country in a concentrated effort.
   When this happens we will see a speed-up in diminishing the accident problem. The organization should investigate the use of a professional fund-raising staff to enlist the support of the public. Probably an
all-out effort of this type could be supported entirely by private and public

   [8] Reprinted courtesy of The Association for the Aid of Crippled Children from
Herbert H. Jacobs's article, "Conceptual and Methodological Problems in Accident
Research," in *Behavioral Approaches to Accident Research* (New York: Ganis and
Harris, 1961), p. 5.

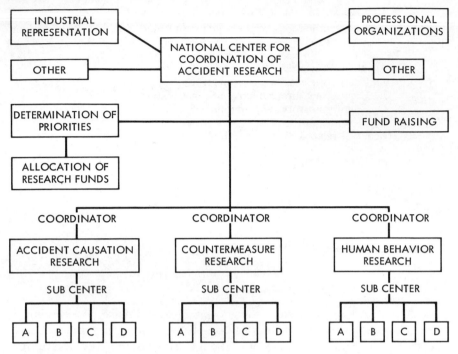

Figure 15-1. *A model for nationwide coordination of accident research.*

funds contributed by individuals, industries and interested organizations. A study of the polio foundation and other voluntary organizations supports this conclusion. Since the National Foundation could raise funds in the neighborhood of 50 to 75 million dollars per year some twenty years ago, the possibilities should be even greater today for a social problem of much more significance.

SUMMARY

Determining the origin of accidents is a very complex problem. The approach to accident research therefore must be multi-disciplined. Because of the many variables in the causes of accidents, their solutions call for efforts from many professions. The approach should be well balanced and well coordinated.

The voluminous nature of past research and the extensiveness of present projects indicate that we need research into the nature and scope of accident research itself. We must assess our present status in accident

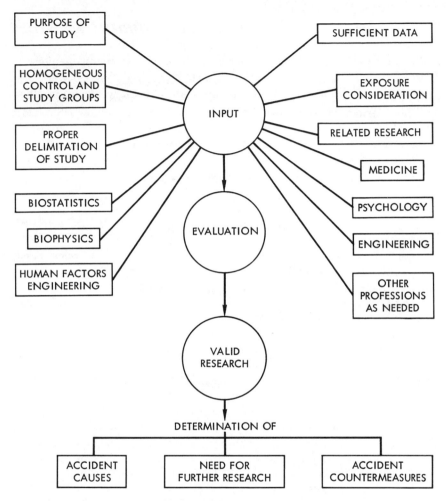

Figure 15-2. *A model for a coordinated research project.*

research and plan for future research needs. Because of the wide scope of accident research, we need a national center to coordinate it.

Our educational programs concerning accidents need reevaluation and redesigning to enlist public support. Experience in areas such as polio indicates that people will respond when they understand the need. If properly educated, the public will contribute the necessary funds and energy to reduce the accident problem dramatically. The answer will not come overnight, but research is the only avenue we can logically follow to find accident causes and workable countermeasures.

SUGGESTED STUDENT ACTIVITIES

1. Design a research project for a selected phase of accident prevention.
2. Write a paper suggesting how a nationwide fund-raising campaign for accident research might serve as a tool for mass education in accident prevention.
3. Write a paper showing how three selected disciplines might enter into a corporate research project.
4. Do a research project to determine some areas where we have good accident-related research.
5. Design a classification system for accident research.

BIBLIOGRAPHY

DRIESSEN, GERALD. "The Fallacy of the Untrained Driver." *Traffic Safety Magazine*, March 1969, p. 17.

HADDON, WILLIAM, JR.; SUCHMAN, EDWARD A.; AND KLEIN, DAVID. *Accident Research, Methods and Approaches.* Association for the Aid of Crippled Children. New York: Harper & Row, 1964.

JACOBS, HERBERT H. "Conceptual and Methodological Problems in Accident Research." In *Behavioral Approaches to Accident Research.* Association for the Aid of Crippled Children. New York: Ganis and Harris, 1961.

KING, B. G. "Some Comments on Accident Prevention Research." *Traffic Safety Research Review* 7 (June 1963), pp. 19–21.

RECHT, J. L. *Systems Safety Analysis: A Modern Approach to Safety Problems.* Special publication. Chicago: National Safety Council, n.d.

SUCHMAN, EDWARD A. "A Conceptual Analysis of the Accident Phenomenon." In *Behavioral Approaches to Accident Research.* Association for the Aid of Crippled Children. New York: Ganis and Harris, 1961.

index